W9-BBT-607

Date: 6/10/19

INFERTILITY TREATMENTS

Recent Titles in Health and Medical Issues Today

Alcohol
Peter L. Myers and Richard E. Isralowitz

Geriatrics
Carol Leth Stone

Plastic Surgery
Lana Thompson

Birth Control
Aharon W. Zorea

Bullying
Sally Kuykendall, PhD

Steroids
Aharon W. Zorea

Suicide and Mental Health
Rudy Nydegger

Cutting and Self-Harm
Chris Simpson

Discrimination against the Mentally Ill
Monica A. Joseph

Concussions
William Paul Meehan III

Drug Resistance
Sarah E. Boslaugh

Work-Life Balance
Janice Arenofsky

The Body Size and Health Debate
Christine L. B. Selby

Obesity: Second Edition
Evelyn B. Kelly

Infertility Treatments

Janice Arenofsky

Health and Medical Issues Today

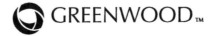

An Imprint of ABC-CLIO, LLC

Santa Barbara, California • Denver, Colorado

Library of Congress Cataloging-in-Publication Data

Names: Arenofsky, Janice, author.
Title: Infertility treatments / Janice Arenofsky.
Description: Santa Barbara, California : Greenwood, [2018] | Series: Health and
    medical issues today | Includes bibliographical references and index.
Identifiers: LCCN 2018008270 (print) | LCCN 2018010806 (ebook) | ISBN
    9781440858864 (ebook) | ISBN 9781440858857 (hard copy : alk. paper)
Subjects: | MESH: Reproductive Techniques, Assisted | Infertility—therapy
Classification: LCC RC889 (ebook) | LCC RC889 (print) | NLM WQ 208 |
    DDC 616.6/9206—dc23
LC record available at https://lccn.loc.gov/2018008270

ISBN: 978–1–4408–5885–7 (print)
        978–1–4408–5886–4 (ebook)

22 21 20 19 18   1 2 3 4 5

This book is also available as an eBook.

Greenwood
An Imprint of ABC-CLIO, LLC

ABC-CLIO, LLC
130 Cremona Drive, P.O. Box 1911
Santa Barbara, California 93116-1911
www.abc-clio.com

This book is printed on acid-free paper ∞

Manufactured in the United States of America

To all the faceless individuals and couples struggling with infertility:
May you reach your desired destinations trusting science
and technology to take you on new pathways.

To my sisters-to-come in the year 2070: Many small steps for women's
reproduction, a giant leap for mankind.

CONTENTS

SERIES FOREWORD

Every day, the public is bombarded with information on developments in medicine and health care. Whether it is on the latest techniques in treatment or research, or on concerns over public health threats, this information directly affects the lives of people more than almost any other issue. Although there are many sources for understanding these topics—from Web sites and blogs to newspapers and magazines—students and ordinary citizens often need one resource that makes sense of the complex health and medical issues affecting their daily lives.

The Health and Medical Issues Today series provides just such a one-stop resource for obtaining a solid overview of the most controversial areas of health care in the twenty-first century. Each volume addresses one topic and provides a balanced summary of what is known. These volumes provide an excellent first step for students and lay people interested in understanding how health care works in our society today.

Each volume is broken into several parts to provide readers and researchers with easy access to the information they need:

- Part I provides overview chapters on background information—including chapters on such areas as the historical, scientific, medical, social, and legal issues involved—that a citizen needs to intelligently understand the topic.
- Part II provides capsule examinations of the most heated contemporary issues and debates, and analyzes in a balanced manner the viewpoints held by various advocates in the debates.
- Part III provides case studies that show examples of the concepts discussed in the previous parts.

A selection of reference material, such as a timeline of important events and a directory of organizations, serves as the best next step in learning about the topic at hand.

The Health and Medical Issues Today series strives to provide readers with all the information needed to begin making sense of some of the most important debates going on in the world today. The series includes volumes on such topics as stem-cell research, obesity, gene therapy, alternative medicine, organ transplantation, mental health, and more.

Although there are worse infirmities than infertility, to those receiving that diagnosis, it is a humbling, distressing experience that can wreck marriages and careers, send self-esteem plummeting, and topple plans for family building. In denial, many people spend years trying to conceive naturally although the medical definition of infertility is only one year of intercourse without attaining a pregnancy. On the other hand, some people go to the other extreme—they panic after six months of negative pregnancy tests and rush to the fertility doctor for answers and assistance.

Sometimes those answers and medical protocols are clear and can be remedied through hormones, surgery, or even weight loss, but other times the reason for infertility is never completely understood—either through clinical tests or through medical history. An unknown cause is a fierce enemy to infertile people. It discombobulates them because they worry that this embarrassing turn of events forever dooms them to the unhappy, stigmatized state of childlessness.

Yet science has kept pace with infertility problems. In the past few decades since the famous 1978 "test-tube" birth of Louise Brown in England, biological innovations have rescued many people from the prognosis of sterility. No longer does infertility limit couples to adoption or the childless option; instead, infertility has become a genetic adventure and a booming industry complete with donor sperm and oocytes, surrogate mothers, and high-tech procedures going by initialisms like ICSI, AI, GIFT, ZIFT, IUD, and IVF. Medical techniques and genome mapping have joined forces to dispense hope to many people whose biological clocks have essentially stopped or failed to function; the LBGT population with their missing gametes; those struggling with infectious diseases like hepatitis B and C, HIV, and Zika; and savior siblings created from a combination of IVF (in vitro fertilization) and PGD (preimplantation genetic diagnosis).

Medical harvesting of sperm and eggs can now return the reproductive function to people made infertile by cancer chemotherapy and those whose spouses or partners have died before family planning had been completed. And because the United States has imposed few regulations on the lucrative fertility industry, physicians compete and can command heavy fees. Their clinics post success rates of live births online at the CDC (Centers for Disease Control and Prevention) website, many of them boasting of high rates due partially to implanting multiples of twos and threes in the uteruses of their patients. For despite the documented danger of multiple births, which have been corroborated by professional societies, patients still agree to multiple implantings because they cannot afford to keep repeating expensive IVF procedures.

With about 500 fertility clinics throughout the United States—and despite a recent trend toward consolidation—there is no shortage of expertise in baby making; the shortage is in patient affordability since unlike other countries, few private health insurance companies or public agencies in the United States provide coverage for infertility (90 percent of IVF occurs abroad). Only 15 states mandate insurance coverage, but they are neither comprehensive nor uniform in their packages. Some people are lucky enough to work for an employer that includes IVF treatments as a perk in their healthcare policy, but in general most Americans must depend on savings accounts, loans from banks or relatives, or mortgage their homes to afford costly treatments. Other individuals may look outside the United States and travel to distant countries like Argentina, Brazil, and India for more affordable fertility treatments. Medical tourism is on the upswing, but while many foreign clinics follow high professional standards, stories of malpractice and incompetence circulate.

This book, *Infertility Treatments*, is organized into three parts. Part I gives an overview of the science and history behind ART (assisted reproductive technology), its global and holistic appeal, its economic and legal ramifications, and the health-related consequences of various fertility procedures. Chapter 1 explains the male and female causes of infertility and describes in some detail the medical treatments (such as artificial insemination and IVF). Gestational surrogacy is discussed as well as the history of ART. Chapter 2 tells how to find and evaluate a fertility center, describes PGD and reproductive tourism, and presents special sections on adoption and alternative fertility therapies that patients can use separately or in conjunction with ART. Chapter 3 describes the average U.S. market value of ART procedures, the states that offer mandated insurance, and the out-of-pocket costs for most people. Chapter 4 gives an overview of some of the state legislation that evolved from court cases related to surrogacy and parentage. Chapter 5 presents the downsides of ART—the health risks to parents and children, such as postpartum depression, birth defects, autism, and leukemia.

Part II discusses the controversies that surround fertility treatments as well as the complications and consequences. Chapter 6 addresses the social and emotional stigma of ART and surrogacy; how women and men cope with it through counseling, support groups, and e-therapy; and how employment can help or hurt. Chapter 7 summarizes the attitudes of different religions regarding infertility treatments, and Chapters 8 and 9 discuss the ethics of ART as they affect parents and children. Chapter 8 describes the ethical four pillars and how they are applied to surrogacy, the number of IVF cycles, eSET versus DET (single embryo transfer versus multiple embryo transfer), posthumous harvesting, and human reproductive cloning. Chapter 9 explores the ethics of the older parental ages for ART, disability rights, child treatment, and the ethics of newer technologies such as mitochondrial replacement therapy (MRT), CRISPR, and next generation sequencing (NGS). Chapter 10 explains the current role of the savior sibling, whose umbilical stem cells can cure a family member's genetic problem and help return a child to good health. Also included is a discussion based on the research of Stanford professor Henry T. Greeley, author of *The End of Sex*, of a reproductive future that includes "Easy PGD" and stem cells.

Part III presents case studies that illustrate key issues related to infertility treatments. A directory of sources for further information, a timeline, and a glossary defining terms that may be unfamiliar to readers have also been included at the end of this book.

Acknowledgments

I wish to express thanks to the national organizations persevering for mandatory infertility insurance coverage in all the 50 states.

I especially want to thank Henry T. Greely, author of *The End of Sex and the Future of Human Reproduction,* for his pithy e-mail explanations of the genetic wizardry of Easy PGD, particularly regarding the "savior sibling." As the Deane F. and Kate Edelman Johnson Professor of Law and Professor of Genetics at Stanford University, Greely predicts a pipeline of reproductive possibilities that will surely astound as well as challenge upcoming generations.

PART I

Overview and Background Information

CHAPTER 1

Infertility and ART (Assisted Reproductive Technology)

The Centers for Disease Control and Prevention (CDC) defines infertility as a medical condition occurring when a man and woman have unprotected sexual intercourse for at least one year and it does not result in a pregnancy. What the CDC omits, however, is the emotional chaos that usually accompanies an infertility diagnosis. Even people who are not particularly passionate about children feel a sense of loss when they discover their body has betrayed them. They may feel unfairly singled out—an oddity among a nation of fertile citizens who can reproduce whenever the spirit moves them.

Nothing could be further from the truth, however. Infertility is all too common, with 50,000 new cases each year in the United States alone. In numbers it rivals diseases like leukemia, pancreatic cancer, and liver cancer. Eleanor Stevenson, a professor at Duke University School of Nursing, says the rate of infertility is higher than that of diabetes.

According to the CDC, 7.3 million American women aged 15–44—or 1 in 10 women—have used fertility services at some time. Grouped under the umbrella term of ART, or assisted reproductive technology, modern fertility treatments entail a complicated series of steps including hormone shots, blood tests, ultrasounds, checkups for cervical mucus, male masturbation, egg harvesting, and much more.

Despite the complex steps and discomfort, especially for women, ART has resulted in more than 500,000 in vitro births between 1985 and 2006. Why is such a risky ordeal so popular? For many people, life is not meaningful without a child, and they will do anything to improve their fertility and chances of conception.

This chapter summarizes those female and male causes of and cures for infertility. It also gives the history of various medical remedies and explains the special circumstances under which ART is used, such as post-humous fertilization and conception after cancer and chemotherapy.

COMMON CAUSES OF FEMALE INFERTILITY

Endometriosis

Endometriosis occurs when uterine tissue is produced outside the uterus and in other organs. Women still menstruate, but tissue outside the uterus travels within the body and causes internal bleeding, pain and inflammation, adhesions, and, for many women, infertility. A relatively common problem, endometriosis occurs when bits of the uterine lining can slough off and block the fallopian tubes or the ovaries. Doctors estimate that 5–10 percent of women of reproductive age have endometriosis. Sometimes, endometriosis can be treated by laparoscopic surgery to remove the misplaced endometrium.

Fibroid Tumors

These are benign growths that strike one of every four women. They can appear inside the uterus and decrease fertility by sometimes causing miscarriages. A new procedure that shrinks fibroids and has a low complication rate is called uterine fibroid embolization (UFE). It blocks the blood flow and growth of the fibroid by injecting small particles called Gelfoam into the blood vessels in the fibroid. A partial UFE, which blocks only the fibroid's small arterial branches, has an even lower complication rate and a higher pregnancy rate of live births. Women who have undergone UFE can then use fertility medication or receive in vitro fertilization (IVF) (Baron et al., *Radiology*, September 2012) to stimulate ovarian production of eggs.

Polycystic Ovary Syndrome

This hormonal disorder often affects ovulation and conception. Usually accompanied by an overproduction of androgens (male hormones) and irregular menstrual cycles, polycystic ovary syndrome (PCOS) sometimes causes women to experience insulin resistance. In 2007, a clinic at John Radcliffe Hospital in Oxford, England, became the first facility to surgically retrieve follicles from the ovaries, place them into a hormone broth for a few days, and then use them in IVF. This process is known as in vitro maturation and is better suited to women with polycystic ovaries for whom hyperstimulating hormones could pose a danger. Nowadays, more than 10 clinics in the United States offer this procedure, according to Henry T. Greely in *The End of Sex* (Harvard University Press, 2016), and it is considered safe.

Primary Ovarian Insufficiency

Known as premature ovarian failure, or POF, this condition results in a loss of ovarian function in women under age 40. Women experience a rise in the follicle-stimulating hormone (FSH) and a diminishing in estrogen. They occasionally get their period, which accounts for the fact that 5–10 percent of these women conceive naturally. POF occurs in 1 in 1,000 women between the ages of 15 and 29 and 1 in 100 women between the ages of 30 and 39. The average age of early onset is 27 years. A family history of POF is linked in about 4 percent of the women experiencing the condition.

Tubal Factor Infertility

This is either complete or partial blockage or scarring of the fallopian tubes. Infertility occurs due to complications in egg gathering, transport, and fertilization or embryo transport to the uterus where implantation is supposed to take place. Tubal factor infertility can come from pelvic inflammatory disease, which is usually caused from exposure to sexually transmitted infections like gonorrhea or chlamydia.

Insufficient Luteal Phase

This happens when the endometrium is inadequately prepared either due to the low production of progesterone in the ovary or because the endometrium does not respond to the progesterone.

Weight

Weight gain can interfere with embryonic implantation. When women achieve weight losses by diet, lifestyle, or bariatric surgery, pregnancy rates and births can increase significantly. Also, the menstrual pattern is more regular, and the numbers of embryos for transfer increase. Furthermore, the numbers of ART cycles that achieve pregnancy are reduced with a decrease in miscarriage rates. Health specialists need to advise overweight or obese women to lose weight prior to natural conception or ART (National Nutrient Database for Standard Reference, 2014).

LESS COMMON CAUSES OF FEMALE INFERTILITY

These causes include multiple miscarriages, uterine abnormalities (congenital or acquired from infections, surgery, or polyps), cervix issues (the lower part of the uterus), workplace and environmental toxins, delayed childbearing (after age 34, there are fewer eggs and their quality diminishes), older age (women in late 30s and older respond more poorly to fertility drugs and are at increased risk of chromosomally abnormal embryos such as a Down syndrome child), and fallopian tubal impairment (faulty tubes that do not convey ova to the uterus are common in older Hispanic and African American women).

MALE CAUSES OF INFERTILITY

In men aged 15–25, the two most common problems are malformed sperm and varicocele, a condition in which the veins in the testicles are too large, causing the testicles to become too warm and killing or damaging sperm. Sometimes there are no symptoms, but other times they include scrotal swelling, a painless testicle lump, an aching pain, or visibly enlarged veins. Varicocele occurs when the valves inside the veins stop blood from flowing properly, resulting in a blood backup. A varicocelectomy can cure the problem. A same-day procedure, the procedure is done under anesthesia and ties off the veins that cause the back flow of blood ("Reversing Male Infertility," *Ivanhoe*, February 2018).

Sperm Speed

To check for sperm speed, doctors look for hormonal imbalances in thyroid and prolactin (produced by the pituitary gland) and for problems in sperm motility (spontaneous movement), concentration, and shapes. Currently, the American Chemical Society is experimenting with "spermbots" that can assist the movement of sperm through the woman's reproductive tract. Sperm are placed in the female's uterus or cervix ("conception caps" cover the cervix top) where it is protected from acidic vaginal secretions and kept in contact with the cervical mucus. Researchers say that although much more work needs to be done before their technique can undergo clinical trials, it is off to a promising start.

LESS COMMON CAUSES OF MALE INFERTILITY

Included here are mumps, cystic fibrosis, and some diseases like tuberculosis and smallpox; inability to produce sperm; accidents harming the testes; cancer treatments like chemotherapy and Klinefelter's syndrome (a chromosomal disorder where men have an extra X chromosome). Also, according to a 2018 study published in *Proceedings of the National Academy of Sciences*, men who take ibuprofen on a regular basis can develop hypogonadism, a hormonal condition that can cause infertility in men.

Men can use daily doses of antioxidants; vitamins A, B, D, and E; and plant extracts to improve sperm quality and productivity. Among the medicinal plants suggested are *Alpinia galanga*, *Danae racemosa*, and *Aloe vera*. Also, a "black box" attached to a microscope (mentioned in *Fertility and Sterility*) is a new imaging process to choose the best sperm candidates for IVF or intracytoplasmic sperm injection (ICSI).

The rest of this chapter describes how ART developed from its simple beginnings in artificial insemination (AI) to more sophisticated procedures like IVF.

HISTORY OF INFERTILITY REMEDIES AND THE MOST COMMONLY USED PROCEDURES TODAY

Infertility has existed since the beginning of time. Physicians and religious seers devised sociocultural theories and processes to explain this malady and help prevent it.

One of the oldest remedies was to pray to the gods, which is why the Romans lit torches and built fires to honor Diana, the goddess of fertility. In the fifteenth century, other theories emerged, which equated childlessness with the work of witches. Another popular theory was that too much sex or not the right type prevented conception. For a few thousand years, infertile women went to midwives or shamans and drank mule urine, rabbit blood, or other concoctions; they often kissed trees, slid on stones, and bathed themselves in special waters.

By 1694, textbooks declared that conception depended on the mixing of fluids produced during orgasm. This put even more stress on couples, who in the 1800s signed up for a brand of infertility treatment called electrotherapy that James Graham of Philadelphia developed. Graham believed women needed sexual pleasure to conceive.

By 1844, the idea of necessitating a female orgasm was eliminated when Frederick Hollick began giving educational lectures about the female anatomical system. This era saw the birth of reproductive surgery's crude surgical attempts to fix the female organs. Dr. J. Marion Sims operated on hundreds of women at the Woman's Hospital in New York, the first U.S. medical facility devoted entirely to feminine complaints. Surgeons removed ovaries or clipped cervixes to fix what they believed were the purely physical blockages to reproduction. Unfortunately, however, most of these so-called cures failed until artificial insemination was practiced.

Artificial Livestock Insemination

Around 1938, Russian researchers began studying AI in domestic farm animals such as cattle and horses. In that same year, E. J. Perry, a New Jersey dairyman, organized AI cooperatives for dairy cows. Meanwhile, rabbit experiments proliferated. In 1934, Gregory Pincus, a Harvard biologist, removed an egg from the ovary of a female rabbit, fertilized it with a salt solution, and then transferred it to the uterus of a second rabbit, which served as an incubator. This was the first animal IVF.

In the next two decades, scientists experimented with different fertility solutions to enhance conception: Several investigators used egg yolk to protect bull sperm cells from temperature shock. Then egg yolk with sodium citrate was added, which increased the viability of semen at five degrees centigrade for up to three days. Next, glycerol was introduced into the extended media (a mixture of skim milk, lactose monohydrate, and other materials) to freeze fowl and bull sperm. Antibiotics also became part of the sperm solution, and one scientist used glycerol to preserve human sperm and store it with solid carbon dioxide as a refrigerant. These advances led to a Chinese scientist combining rabbit eggs and sperm in a flask for three to four hours in 1959 and producing several four-cell embryos he nurtured into healthy female rabbits.

Artificial Human Insemination

According to the historical documents of Belgian gynecologist Willem Ombelet and American bioethicist Whitny Braun, AI in humans dates back at least to the late eighteenth century when a London physician injected a husband's semen into his wife's vagina with a syringe. The woman became pregnant and later gave birth to a healthy child. In 1790, the experiment appeared in a medical journal.

In the 1850s, American surgeon J. Marion Sims reported his findings of postcoital tests and 55 inseminations performed on African American women in Alabama. Only one pregnancy occurred, probably due to bad timing and the mistaken belief that ovulation occurred during menstruation. In 1884, Dr. William Pancoast, at Jefferson Medical College in Philadelphia, treated an infertile Quaker couple. Pancoast believed infertility was due to this man's blocked seminal ducts from gonorrhea acquired years earlier. Pancoast performed an ethically debatable experiment, inseminating the wife with the sperm from one of Pancoast's most attractive medical students after anesthetizing the wife with chloroform and inserting the semen with a rubber syringe. The wife delivered a healthy baby boy.

Hysterosalpingography

Fallopian tubes received attention in 1917 through a method known as hysterosalpingography that flushes the tubes with iodized poppy seed oil or dye. Doctors injected these liquids during an X-ray scan to check for blockages. This procedure made a comeback in 2017 when used on 1,119 women at the University of Adelaide (*Science Daily*. "100-Year-Old Fertility Technique Reduces Need for IVF," May 18, 2017). Some women got poppy seed oil; others got water. Of those who received the poppy seed oil, 40 percent got pregnant over the next six months compared with 29 percent of those who received water. Researchers do not yet know why the procedure has such an effect, but ultrasounds are gradually eliminating the potentially unsafe use of X-rays. Doctors recommend hysterosalpingography before undergoing IVF. Side effects can include pelvic pain, a small amount of vaginal bleeding, fever, or chills.

Intrauterine Insemination in Humans

The history of intrauterine insemination (IUI) or AI goes back to the eighteenth century when Scottish surgeon John Hunter performed an effective procedure with the use of a husband's sperm. In 1884, after William Pankhurst from Philadelphia applied the donor's sperm, a live birth was reported, and it was noted that placing sperm in a woman's vagina or cervix when she is ovulating sometimes succeeds. The sperm travel into the fallopian tubes to fertilize the woman's egg or eggs. IUI can be done within a clinical or home environment and has no known negative side effects. Also, the flushing is a fraction of the cost of one cycle of IVF, so researchers suggest the "turkey baster" method of flushing prior to opting for IVF.

A semen sample for the baster is collected through masturbation or a collection condom, and a chemical known as a cryoprotectant is added to the sample, which is called the "washed sperm." The washing involves several processes to make the sperm more similar to the normal condition of sperm when it reaches the vagina. Washing also removes potentially problematic components of the semen usually left in the vagina in normal intercourse and helps remove sexually transmitted viruses like HIV and Hepatitis. The semen is then mixed with a nutrient-rich fluid and centrifuged or spun very rapidly for five minutes.

For best results, AI, which has a low success rate, is normally carried out after the woman has ovulated so that ultrasound and/or blood tests are used to monitor her cycle. At that time, the sperm is inserted directly into the uterus with a fine catheter. A speculum keeps the vagina open so the catheter can pass through the cervix into the uterus. The procedure is painless and quick, and the doctor may ask the woman to lie down for a few minutes afterward to let the sperm settle into her body.

When an IUI is conducted at home, a woman self-inseminates with a man's sperm using a syringe or other injectable device to shoot the sperm into her body. At-home procedures can be medically risky as the sperm is not washed. The source of the sperm can be from the intended father, an anonymous or known donor, or a blended mix. Blending can help increase the success rate if the intended father has a low sperm count.

IUI theoretically increases the number of sperm that reach the fallopian tubes and subsequently increases the chance of fertilization.

In Vitro Fertilization

Dr. Kenneth Gelman, who practices ART in Florida, says that IVF, which mixes gametes in a Petri dish and then implants them in the uterus, doubles the success rate compared to IUI. In the 1950s and 1960s, when Dr. Robert Edwards was researching IVF, he was so afraid of criticism for creating human life in a Petri dish that he destroyed the evidence and kept his research a secret. Not until British doctor Patrick Steptoe joined forces with Edwards in 1978 did the creation of the first human pregnancy through IVF take place.

The British couple Lesley and John Brown desperately wanted a child, but Lesley's fallopian tubes were blocked from uterine scarring. Steptoe and Edwards introduced the two gametes—sperm and egg—into a Petri dish and transferred the fertilized embryo into Lesley's uterus. The embryo implanted, and Lesley became pregnant. On July 25, 1978, Dr. Steptoe performed a cesarean section and delivered the first "test tube baby."

Since that first birth, researchers have experimented with forms of IVF termed traditional, conventional, or mild. The variations relate to the use of different amounts of fertility medications, but the same six steps take place: first, the woman receives ovarian stimulation through hormonal injections; next, egg retrieval is conducted (the goal is 8–10 eggs); then comes the fertilization of the egg and sperm (about 50 percent of eggs will fertilize and half will develop into embryos); and the embryos are transferred into the uterus. If they are not transferred, they undergo cryopreservation or freezing. Lastly, the woman gets a pregnancy test.

See Chapter 3 for information on the average costs of IVF and other ART procedures.

Traditional IVF

With traditional IVF, injectable hormones are used to maximize the number of eggs retrieved, increase the number of embryos, and facilitate the selection of the healthiest embryo(s) for transfer. The advantages are more eggs, more embryos, a better pregnancy rate with good responders, and an increased possibility for embryo cryopreservation (freezing and storage) for future use. The disadvantages are cost, multiple monitoring visits, many drug injections, an increased number of eggs (a problem if you want or need only a few), increased risk of OHSS or ovarian hyperstimulation syndrome (a medical condition that can range from mild to serious, affecting the ovaries of some women who take fertility medications to stimulate egg growth), and the need for more anesthesia during egg retrieval due to multiple vaginal needle probes.

In an April 2014 study based on the data from the American National IVF Registry, results from 256,381 IVF cycles revealed the physiological burden that traditional IVF can impose on women. Results showed that the retrieval of more than 15 eggs significantly increases the risk of OHSS without improving live birth rates. A second study in June 2015 showed that women who produced 66,539 singletons from IVF and had 15 eggs collected had a significantly higher chance of having a low birth weight and preterm baby. The outcomes of both these studies suggest that an elevated estrogen level created by higher hormone doses can have a detrimental effect on mother and offspring.

Geeta Nargund, medical director of CREATE Fertility in the United Kingdom and a proponent of natural and mild IVF, believes that the British Human Fertilisation and Embryology Authority needs to collect data about the drugs given to women, especially since clinics currently compete for success rates per cycle. Women need to weigh events in clinics other than success rates before choosing a clinic—such as adverse incidents like OHSS, low birth weight, stillbirth, and prematurity. This can help them make more balanced decisions regarding clinics.

Natural IVF

This process was used to conceive the first "test tube" baby, Louise Joy Brown. It releases one egg during a woman's normal monthly cycle, and then collects and fertilizes it. Today, natural IVF is used when women want to avoid taking ovarian-stimulating drugs with their negative side effects. Gonadotropins (gonad-stimulating hormone) in the hypothalamus gland of the brain initiates natural mechanisms in the pituitary to release FSH, luteinizing hormone (LH), estrogen, and progesterone. No drugs are used for ovarian hyperstimulation, but they may be used for ovulation suppression, after which the eggs are released, harvested, frozen, and transferred to the uterus in a later natural cycle.

According to a study of 1,503 modified natural IVF cycles in the *Journal of Assisted Reproduction and Genetics* (Shaulov, July 2015), this procedure is considered an acceptable treatment option for women 35 years old and younger and for women 36 years and older with normal ovarian responses.

Mild IVF

According to Geeta Nargund, the difference between natural IVF and mild IVF is that in the former, the egg is automatically selected by the woman's ovary and the process involves no stimulating drugs. Mild IVF, however, involves the use of low doses of drug stimulation for five to nine days in the woman's natural menstrual cycle. By avoiding the use of a high number of drugs, the possibility of OHSS is lessened as well as some of the physical and psychological discomforts, side effects, and risks. Furthermore, the total cost is less, and scientific evidence shows that the lining of the uterus is healthier for implantation.

The birth weight of babies born from mild IVF is higher compared with traditional IVF, so it is a win-win situation for both mother and child. Mild IVF also can be used in which a small dose of ovarian-stimulating drugs is used during a woman's natural cycle. The aim is to produce two to seven eggs, some of which when fertilized will develop into healthy embryos. This method reduces complications and side effects and is aimed at the quality of eggs and embryos, not quantity. Mild IVF can also be cheaper than traditional IVF and reduce the risk of multiple births. Egg retrieval is usually done by transvaginal ultrasound aspiration in the doctor's office. A man's sperm and a woman's egg are combined in a laboratory dish, and one or more fertilized embryos can be transferred into the woman's uterus for implantation.

IVF Ovulation Drugs

According to the website WebMD, Clomid and Serophene (brand names of clomiphene) are the two most commonly prescribed fertility drugs. If Clomid does not work by itself, physicians may recommend other hormones such as human chorionic gonadotropin (hCG), FSH, human menopausal gonadotropin (hMG), gonadotropin-releasing hormone (GnRH), and GnRH agonist. Some are given beneath the skin or subcutaneously, while others are injected into the muscle. Injections can be in the stomach, upper arm, upper thigh, or buttocks.

About 60–80 percent of women who take clomiphene will ovulate and about half will get pregnant. Most pregnancies happen within three cycles. Women who use clomiphene citrate also have approximately a 5–8 percent chance of having twins. Studies show that pregnancy rates with aromatase inhibitors are similar to clomiphene citrate rates and can be better used in certain ovulation disorders like PCOS.

Gonadotropins containing FSH or LH or a combination of the two drugs may be prescribed for women who have tried clomiphene citrate without conceiving. The goal is to attain one or more mature follicles and an appropriate estrogen level so ovulation can be triggered by hCG (this mimics the natural LH surge and causes the dominant follicle to release its egg and ovulate).

The potential risk and complications include multiple pregnancy, premature delivery, and negative health consequences for the newborn such as breathing problems, bleeding in the brain, cerebral palsy, infections, and death. Side effects for women include breast tenderness, abdominal bloating, mild abdominal pain, and mood swings.

Less-Used IVF Techniques
Assisted Zona Hatching

Carried out shortly before the embryo transfer, a small opening is made in the outer layer surrounding the egg (the zona pellucida [ZP]) to help the embryo hatch out and aid in the implantation process. In some women, the ZP becomes toughened, restricting the embryo from hatching so assisted hatching helps the embryo exit its protective "shell" and implant into the uterine lining. Numerous studies have shown that *this* improves pregnancy and implantation rates. The most common scenarios for implementing assisted hatching with IVF are the following:

- Women over 38 years and using their own eggs
- Women with repeated failure of embryo implantation
- Women whose embryos exhibit thick ZP
- Women with elevated FSH levels
- Women with poor embryo quality

Intracytoplasmic Sperm Injection

In 1993, Sherman Spielberg and his colleagues performed ICSI, which enhanced male fertility by injecting a single sperm into an egg and achieving fertilization. The technique developed from the late 1980s' work in Australia on injecting sperm into the egg's ZP. In ICSI, a microscope-guided needle gets hold of a single sperm, breaks its tail, and injects it directly into the egg. Doctors use tiny needles and micromanipulators (tools that lessen the hand's movement). This produces much higher rates of fertilization than earlier methods. ICSI greatly increases the probability of producing pregnancies from men with very low sperm counts or with dysfunctional sperm.

After masturbation, the man has his semen treated or washed by removing the seminal fluid and nonfunctioning sperm cells. Some single sperm will be picked out for ICSI. Although ICSI was first developed for use for men with fertility problems, it is now used in nearly 70 percent of IVF cycles in the United States (Greely).

Since ICSI's overall pregnancy rates, according to Debora L. Spar in *The Baby Business* (Harvard Business School Press, 2006), are about 32 percent, new fertility centers added this ART tool to their offerings, typically charging $1,000 to $1,500 for the procedure. Unfortunately, according to several studies, male children born via ICSI lack the same gene that their fathers lack, meaning they too are likely to be infertile. Nevertheless, tens of thousands of children were born using ICSI during the 1990s.

Overall pregnancy and delivery rates with ICSI are similar to rates with traditional IVF. In a May 2016 *Science Daily* report on ICSI, 220,000 IVF treatments took place in 2010 and more than 455,000 ICSI procedures. Most patients who get pregnant with ICSI will also do so with IVF.

Gamete Intrafallopian Transfer

The American Society for Reproductive Medicine (ASRM) describes two common ART processes that are variations of IVF. In gamete intrafallopian transfer (GIFT), gametes (egg and sperm) are transferred to the woman's fallopian tubes rather than to her uterus, and fertilization takes place in the tubes rather than in a laboratory Petri dish. The use of laparoscopy—a surgical procedure that may be necessary to transfer the gametes to the tubes—is often part of the protocol.

GIFT is only for women with normal fallopian tubes. Some couples may prefer GIFT for religious reasons since the eggs are fertilized inside the body. One limitation of GIFT is that fertilization cannot be confirmed immediately as with IVF. Currently, GIFT is carried out in less than 1 percent of ART procedures in the United States. GIFT can be used with women who have at least one healthy fallopian tube, according to the American Pregnancy Association

Zygote Intrafallopian Transfer

In zygote intrafallopian transfer (ZIFT), fertilization takes place in the lab in vitro (outside the body), but the fertilized eggs are then transferred within 24 hours to the fallopian tube rather than to the uterus. This procedure requires a laparoscopy (abdominal surgery performed through a small keyhole-size incision with the aid of an inserted camera) to collect the eggs. ZIFT is carried out in less than 1 percent of ART procedures in the United States.

NEWER VARIATIONS OF ART

Fresh versus Frozen Gametes and Embryos

Cryopreservation began in the 1980s, and since then, experts have debated the pros and cons of frozen versus fresh gametes and embryos. In August 2016, an obstetrician/gynecologist at Penn State University announced the results of his study on women with PCOS, a hormonal disorder that causes enlarged ovaries with small cysts on the outside. He concluded that frozen embryos produced more live births than fresh embryos and may be a preferred treatment for women with PCOS.

Also, according to a July 2015 report, doctors say that the new quick-freeze method preserves the IVF success rate at the age at which the eggs are frozen. Frozen eggs behave like fresh ones, and initial studies show no increased risk of birth defects. However, as with any medical procedure, risks are associated with egg freezing. Among them are ovarian torsions—a condition in which a woman's ovaries twist and balloon to the size of grapefruits and forces the woman to go to the emergency room to have her ovaries drained. Despite this risk, Gina Bartasi, founder and CEO of EggBanxx and now the head of the fertility company Progyny, estimates that by 2018, 76,000 UK women will freeze their eggs every year.

The statistics regarding fresh versus frozen embryos yielding live births can be confusing, but law and genetics professor Henry T. Greely (*The End of Sex*) says recent trials of frozen embryos of good quality seem to be more successful than the fresh ones, perhaps because freezing gives the prospective mother's reproductive system time to return to the norm from the hormones used in IVF.

Gestational Surrogacy

Not long after the "test tube" birth of Louise Joy Brown came a raft of pregnancies and births from egg donations where the surrogate mother was not the genetic mother. Those early cases around 1983, according to Greely, involved women who could not produce viable eggs but could manage pregnancies using donated eggs.

Nowadays, gestational surrogacy is used for most of the surrogacy cycles in the United States. The woman carries a baby conceived using the egg of the intended mother or an egg donor and sperm from the intended father or a sperm donor. Gestational surrogacy is a good option for women with thin endometrial linings, recurrent uterine fibroids, congenital uterine abnormalities, an absent uterus, or multiple failed IVF cycles. It has become the procedure of choice for couples, singles, same-sex couples, and women with medical problems. Prospective parents choose donors based in part on donors' physical and intellectual characteristics. They can afford to be picky about sperm because men produce many gametes while egg brokers typically have much smaller inventories of oocytes available.

According to the Society for Assisted Reproductive Technology (SART), over 1,000 babies are born annually in the United States via gestational or commercial surrogacy. In commercial surrogacy, a surrogate receives a base compensation for carrying the intended parents' child in addition to reimbursement for all pregnancy-related costs. Commercial surrogacy can be a complicated legal and ethical matter, as some state laws do not allow for compensated surrogacy of any kind. In most of the United States, surrogacy laws permit surrogacy contracts, grant pre-birth orders, and name both parents on the birth certificate, but some states may prohibit compensated surrogacy or make it impossible for both intended parents to be listed on the child's birth certificate.

Gestational surrogacy is legally simpler because the surrogate is not biologically related to the child she is carrying since the embryo is created by the intended parents (using a donated sperm or egg if necessary) and then transferred to the surrogate's uterus. Surrogates are only reimbursed for pregnancy-related costs.

Because surrogacy is illegal in five states in the United States and in many countries (such as Canada and the United Kingdom), only 571 surrogacy contracts were reported in 2001. Since agencies are not required to report surrogate births, data are limited, but statistics from the SART show a dramatic increase in surrogate births over the past decade—up from 738 in 2004 to 2,236 in 2014.

Some intended parents choose altruistic surrogacy, where a surrogate, usually a friend or relative, does not receive any additional compensation beyond the coverage of pregnancy-related costs. Embryos are fertilized outside the womb through IVF and then implanted, or transferred, into the surrogate's uterus where it remains until delivery. Kirsten Langhammer is such a surrogate. She gave birth to three sets of twins for three couples in the past four years (*St. Louis Post-Dispatch*, May 2016). Although the real estate worker said it had been a "positive" experience, not everybody in her own family agrees.

Infection-Less Babies

According to the Americans with Disabilities Act (1990), couples with blood-borne viruses like Ebola, Zika, HIV, Hepatitis B, and Hepatitis C must not be denied ART since with minor modifications, these infectious patients can receive safe treatment. Dr. Sangita K. Jindal in her 2016 article in *Reproductive Biomedicine Online* restates the 2014 CDC protocol that says couples in the United States with a positive virus from the male may use IUI, IVF, or ICSI if the semen has been washed and thus rid of the virus. Washing helps improve the ability of sperm to move toward the egg and helps remove sexually transmitted viruses. Couples using donated eggs, sperms, or embryos should follow the infectious precautions outlined by the Food and Drug Administration (FDA) for Zika, Hepatitis, and other infections:

- Reject donations if the donor has had a Zika virus diagnosis in the past six months, has resided in or traveled to an area with active Zika within the past six months, or has had sex with a man within the past six months who was diagnosed with Zika.
- Use gametes or embryos from ineligible donors if the tissue is labeled to indicate higher risk; everyone is aware of and willing to take the risk; and physicians know the status of the eggs, sperm, or embryos.

The World Health Organization (WHO) says that about 5 percent of the population are chronic carriers of Hepatitis B. According to a Hepatitis study in *Women's Health & Gynecology* (April 2016), pregnancy is not contraindicated unless the liver function has been compromised. However, the mother has a 10 percent risk of passing the infection to her child at birth.

Though studies have shown that viral Hepatitis can cause male infertility and a less than optimum response in ART, there are no significant differences in live births when compared with couples without the virus. In fact, benefits exist when using ART due to early intervention with prenatal treatment to reduce transmission to the child. In a 2016 study in which Hepatitis B was involved in 43 cases, researchers found that the Hepatic virus in gametes could have negative effects on fertility and could be transmitted to the fetuses, but sperm washing and ART help prevent that transmission. The study concluded that ART is useful in reducing the risk of Hepatitis B.

IVF as Agent to Combat Cancer Infertility

Assisted reproduction procedures can help cancer patients retain their fertility. Cryopreservation of eggs, sperm, and embryos is the best way. Patients then can undergo surgery, radiation, and chemotherapy and not have to worry about their future reproductive abilities. As long as patients do not expose their developing baby to cancer treatments, children do not appear to be affected by congenital disorders or other health problems.

Posthumous Reproduction

A study of 1,049 U.S. residents in *Fertility and Sterility* (Barton et al., July 2012) showed that almost 50 percent of the population support posthumous reproduction—retrieving sperm and eggs from deceased men and women. This allows a person to conceive a child with someone after that person is deceased. However, the person undergoing ART should consult a lawyer to work out any legal obstacles. In an article on dead soldiers and their posthumously conceived children in the 2014 *Journal of Contemporary Health Law and Policy*, the author describes how the decision to harvest sperm or eggs from a deceased or incompetent person has implications for inheritance, estate planning, will drafting, trusts, Social Security claims, child support, and custody issues.

Most people favor prior consent from the deceased. The European Society of Human Reproduction and Embryology (ESHRE) has guidelines on emergency requests for sperm or egg retrieval, which the ASRM accepted in June 2013. In the absence of written consent from the deceased, requests for posthumous gamete retrieval or reproduction should only be honored if the requests are initiated by the surviving spouse or life partner.

CONCLUSION

This chapter dealt with the medical reasons and basic techniques underlying the use of ART. Most ART procedures are IVF-related whether the eggs, sperms, and embryos are from donors or from prospective parents or surrogates. Different fertility drugs are used to initiate maximum ovulation, and side effects can vary from hot flashes, blurred vision, nausea, bloating, and headache to ovarian hyperstimulation.

Related ART procedures are ZIFT, GIFT, ICSI, and gestational and altruistic surrogacy. Gestational surrogacy has increased tremendously in the past decade for legal reasons. At the same time, the use of frozen sperm has increased rather than fresh sperm. People with infectious diseases can also become parents because science and the "washing" of gametes can assist them in reducing their chances of transmitting HIV, Hepatitis B, Hepatitis C, and Zika to their children.

The next chapter focuses on alternatives to choosing the usual IVF route. After examining the factors that determine the rankings of American fertility clinics, readers may wish to switch from the traditional to other options, among which are reproductive tourism, adoption, preimplantation genetic diagnosis (PGD), and alternative fertility therapies such as acupuncture and hypnotherapy.

CHAPTER 2

Growing Families

After more than 40 years, Assisted Reproductive Technology (ART) remains a divisive topic among Americans. A 2013 poll by the Pew Research Center found that 12 percent of Americans think in vitro fertilization (IVF) is wrong; 33 percent find it acceptable; and 46 percent are indifferent. The overarching fear for many Americans is that scientists have opened a Pandora's box of high-tech genetic techniques that will inevitably lead to human cloning, eugenics à la Hitler, and the birth of babies in artificial wombs. Not surprisingly they reject this dystopian *Gattaca-Brave-New-World* vision.

As seen in Chapter 1, some of what people fear most about assisted conception is already taking place, with laboratory technicians combining fresh and frozen eggs and sperm (from donors or intended parents) to form fertilized embryos that are implanted in the woman's uterus. However, attempting to resist scientific progress in baby making is impossible in a free and democratic society. Science and technology have a way of merging their creativity to push us forward into new territory. Progress also is self-defeating since building a family in the old-fashioned way through sex does not work for everyone.

It did not work for Marla B. Neufeld, the author of the *ABA Guide to Assisted Reproduction*. Multiple miscarriages and numerous fertility treatments resulted in protracted frustration. Marla ultimately had to use a gestational surrogate who carried and gave birth to her twin boys.

In this chapter same-gender infertility rates in the United States are also discussed as well as the many choices available to infertile couples, the attributes of top-notch fertility physicians and clinics, alternative and holistic treatments couples may want to try before consenting to ART or in conjunction with it, the adoption option, travel overseas to different countries to receive fertility treatments (medical tourism), and the option to employ preimplantation genetic diagnosis (PGD) to genetically scan for serious diseases.

Nowadays ART, considered one of the top major medical advances in the past 65 years, has changed the way people create families. Couples no longer need to have sexual intercourse to have a child. Mothers can use egg donations to become pregnant, a lesbian or gay couple can invest in gestational surrogacy, and a grief-stricken husband can harvest an oocyte from his dead wife.

INFERTILITY RATES

Infertility is a global condition affecting between 8 percent and 12 percent of reproductive-aged couples worldwide. In some regions the rate of infertility is much higher, reaching 30 percent in areas like South Asia, the Middle East, and central and eastern Europe. In the United States infertility affects about 10 percent to 12 percent of women aged 15–44, according to the National Health Statistics Report of 2013. Henry T. Greely in *The End of Sex* says the use of ART has doubled in the past decade, with 400,000 IVF babies born each year.

Infertility is not gender specific. Males experience it about one-fourth of the time; women, about one-half of the time; and the remaining quarter of cases remain a mystery to medical science. No one knows why certain couples remain infertile. Sometimes only minor abnormalities such as sperm dysfunction occur (which should not result in infertility) but somehow they do.

Depression may play a role. A 2009 study concluded there might be a correlation between infertility of unknown origin and depression, with most adults experiencing their first depressive episode prior to their diagnosis of infertility (*Journal of Psychosomatic Obstetrics & Gynecology*). Along the same lines, a Danish study at the University of Copenhagen concluded that women who give birth after fertility treatments are at higher risk of depression (five times more) than women not bearing a child following fertility treatment. These results from 41,000 women are surprising because until 2015 it was assumed that the reverse was true and women not becoming pregnant would develop depression. These new data shed a different light on ART. Some researchers have now concluded that fertility treatments can be tough even when success arrives.

However, there appears to be a silver lining to fertility treatments even when they fail to produce a pregnancy. In a July 2016 article at the website MedlinePlus, Robert Preidt reported that almost 3 in 10 women get pregnant naturally within two years after their fertility treatment, and there is almost a 30 percent likelihood of conceiving over a six-year period, according to Dr. Samuel Marcus, an obstetrician-gynecologist at Queen Elizabeth Hospital in London. Findings from the Danish IVF Register are similar, concluding that the overall birth rate within five years of initiating fertility treatment was 71 percent among nearly 20,000 women (*Ob Gyn News*, August 2016).

FERTILITY CENTERS

When women seek fertility treatment, they often depend on a reference to a great doctor. They do their due diligence asking friends, relatives and other health professionals and consulting the Centers for Disease Control and Prevention (CDC) "success" website for live births. And it is true— a great doctor can make all the difference, but the not-as-well-known fact is that the doctor's embryology laboratory often drives a lot of that difference between the nearly 500 fertility clinics in the United States. Most are for-profit businesses and are members of Society for Assisted Reproductive Technology (SART), a professional organization of physicians and fertility centers that establish ART standards. They also adhere to the federal 1992 Fertility Clinic Success Rate and Certification Act administered by the CDC, which issues reports on the clinics' success rates with IVF. To find a good laboratory, the CDC success site is your best bet— the quality of the embryology lab is a strong driver of clinic success rates.

However, despite the perceived accuracy of these statistical reports, clinic success rates cannot be regarded as 100 percent valid since their numbers can be easily massaged by clinics eager to attract clients. The statistics for clinics are often presented in a misleading way to enhance the clinics' market value. For example, a clinic's success rate for women aged 41–42 may indicate an 11.2–12.4 percent success rate. While this figure is accurate, the data would have a far different impact if framed as a "failure rate" (which you will never see) because women then would understand that their IVF cycle has almost a 9 in 10 chances of failing. Since many women incorrectly believe that IVF works more often than not, citing the "failure" rate might bring a little more reality into the comparative picture.

(Online information on IVF outcomes is available from SART and the CDC. A new reporting structure debuted in 2016 due to the growing popularity of transferring frozen—not fresh—embryos. People can evaluate a state's clinical report at the States Monitoring ART—SMART— Collaborative, CDC, for the number of successful IVF cycles for fresh, frozen, and donor eggs by the woman's age.)

Another example of positive spinning of data is that some clinics encourage certain patients to drop out of IVF programs earlier. These are usually patients who do not get pregnant within a certain amount of time or those whose follicle-stimulating hormone levels are higher. The clinics are really selecting the best—and easiest—patients to treat, which artificially increases their success rates.

Sean Tipton, a SART spokesperson, says the CDC data are primarily a professional tool for the industry and do not necessarily give infertile couples a good idea of their chances of success. He says SART is working on a free online patient predictor model that gives patients a better sense of clinic success. That being said, the success rate depends on many factors such as maternal age, cause of infertility, embryo status, reproductive history, and lifestyle factors. For instance, younger women are more likely to get pregnant using IVF, and women older than 41 are more likely to get pregnant with a donor egg. Judging by reproductive history, women who have been previously pregnant have more success with IVF than those who have never been pregnant.

The latest data in the Assisted Reproductive Technology National Summary Report (as reported on the CDC website) indicate that in 2014, clinics started 208,604 IVF cycles, 3,596 of which used frozen eggs. These cycles led to different results for different-aged women. For women under age 35, the rate of live births after embryo transfer was about 47 percent; for women aged 35–37, 44 percent; women 38–40, 38 percent; women 41–42, 32 percent; women 43–44, 23 percent; and around 14 percent for women over 44. (For further help understanding success rates, Debora L. Spar's *The Baby Business* [Harvard Business School Press, 2006] includes a chart listing the 20 top fertility clinics in 2002 by the number of IVF cycles carried out.)

Vetting Fertility Clinics

Evaluating fertility clinics is not easy, but a checklist of criteria can be useful. Good fertility clinics have several things in common, says the *ABA Guide to Assisted Reproduction* (ABA, 2016). They invest in state-of-the-art laboratories, do exhaustive patient workups, have multiple stimulation protocols, and conduct egg/sperm transfers that are relatively trauma free.

Also, patients might ask the following:

- What procedures do you offer?
- How much experience do you have?
- What are your criteria—for instance, age or marital status—for accepting new patients?
- What tests are required?
- Do you have a protocol for arranging to obtain or secure donor eggs, embryos, or sperm?
- Do you offer elective single embryo transfer (eSET) or one embryo implant?
- What would be the schedule for the ART procedure I would have?
- What are the costs for storage of eggs, sperm, or embryos?
- What types of counseling and support services are available?
- Are the physician boards certified?
- Are you affiliated with the American Society for Reproductive Medicine (ASRM)?

(Adapted from CDC *Questions to Ask When Selecting an ART Provider or Clinic*, CDC.gov)

PREIMPLANTATION GENETIC DIAGNOSIS

One question that consumers definitely should ask is: Does your clinic carry out PGD? Currently more than 50 clinics around the world, including several in the United States, offer genetic screening of embryo to identify single-gene mutation diseases such as Fanconi anemia, thalassemia, phenylketonuria, and Fragile X Syndrome. (See Chapter 10 for its use with "savior siblings.") Typically, only single-gene mutation diseases are currently identifiable. Gender is also identifiable due to sex-linked diseases such as hemophilia and muscular dystrophy.

As with ART, the United States does not regulate PGD. Instead it has left the decision making up to professional societies such as ASRM and the American College of Medical Genetics, which maintain that children deserve the right to be healthy. For example, although PGD increases the cost of IVF by $4,000–$7,500, the added benefit is the 24 Chromosome Microarray, a $1,500 test that can analyze the entire chromosomal content of embryos. In 2007, about 5 percent of 132,745 IVF procedures in the United States included PGD, according to *Reproductive Technology*; in 2012, 5 percent of the IVF cycles in the United States used PGD, yielding about 3,000 PGD children. PGD is sometimes covered by insurance if it is being used to avoid a known high-risk genetic disease in the child.

The story of PGD can be traced back to the 1930s and agricultural gender experiments. By 1980 scientists began working to identify the gender of early-stage embryos to guard against specific sex-linked diseases. They succeeded in 1989 after scientists identified a couple who both carried the gene for cystic fibrosis from a single cell of an eight-cell embryo (a blastocyst).

However, PGD is neither foolproof nor entirely risk free, which is why some countries regulate it. Different countries permit or disallow some or all of the four specific purposes that PGD is used for: to avoid serious genetic diseases known to run in the family, to select an embryo with immune system genes that make it a possible umbilical cord donor for a sick relative (savior child), to choose gender, and, most commonly, to try to pick embryos that are more likely to survive the implantation and development process and become healthy babies. For example, Germany enacted the Embryo Protection Act of 1990 to prohibit PGD; other countries such as Italy, Switzerland, and France permit PGD, but their governments control its use. Britain's Human Fertilisation and Embryology Authority (HFEA) authorizes only limited use of PGD, allowing sex selection to avoid sex-linked disorders as well as conditions associated with disability or serious medical conditions. Besides children's diseases, PGD can report on the risk levels of embryonic children for adult diseases such as colon cancer, breast cancer, ovarian cancer, and Alzheimer disease.

As an additional safeguard, physicians may test parents who either have the disease or are carriers for simple Mendelian diseases such as cystic fibrosis or Huntington's disease. Greely (*The End of Sex*) says avoiding serious health issues is PGD's mission since it falls within the ethical toolbox of beneficence (producing good) and autonomy (parents or children wanting to prevent serious diseases—see Chapters 8 and 9 for more on ethics). For instance, in 2017 an international team published a study in the *American Journal of Human Genetics* concluding that about 7 percent of gene mutations in parents can lead to the development of autism spectrum disorder in children. These data indicate that physicians should require more sensitive PGD testing of both children and parents.

Gender selection through PGD has been widely practiced in the United States to avoid sex-linked diseases, but when used for social or cultural purpose, it is unethical. It can reinforce sex discrimination, gender stereotyping, and anti-feminism. PGD is also not considered ethical for the selection of eye or hair color since it does not fall into the "right to health" category. One criticism of PGD is that it is dehumanizing since the entire process transfers procreation from the home to the laboratory, transforming birth into a commodity. Another criticism is that not everyone can afford the add-on IVF test. PGD also could make incest not only possible but also safer.

Not a lot of scientific data exist regarding the health results of children born after PGD, but based on anecdotal reports, PGD has not produced a huge number of miscarriages, stillbirths, or neonatal deaths. However, no registry exists to track PGD health risks in children, but mosaicism is a possibility. Every cell is not identical, and the mutations (mosaicism) can be harmless or lead to a serious disease like cancer. Due to mosaicism, parents in the United States who use PGD to assess a possible pregnancy are also encouraged to use prenatal fetal diagnosis (amniocentesis or chorionic villus sampling) later in the pregnancy to double check the PGD fetus.

The main disadvantage of PGD is that it can only be used effectively in conjunction with IVF, which is why its use hovers around 5 percent of births. Widespread use of PGD has to await the time when there is an easier way than IVF to obtain eggs for fertilization (see Chapter 10 and "Easy PGD").

According to Greely, noninvasive prenatal testing, or NIPT, may eventually supersede PGD. NIPT tests the fetus's DNA by finding small pieces in a blood sample drawn from the pregnant woman. NIPT made its first commercial debut in the United States in 2011. Its advantages have made it a highly requested test now offered in over 60 countries with prices rapidly decreasing. Its use has boomed in the United States. By 2015 it was used in several hundred thousand American pregnancies, the majority of them screening for Down syndrome. The cost is between $800 and $2,400 in the United States.

REPRODUCTIVE TOURISM

The United States is a great provider of surrogates, with California and New Jersey leading the way, but many Americans cannot find a fertility facility appropriate for them and their pocketbook due to often confusing state regulations and high costs for IVF and surrogacy. As a result, reproductive tourism—traveling to another country for fertility procedures—has become popular, especially with couples lacking insurance. For example, couples may pay an estimated $50,000 surrogacy fee in the United States whereas surrogacy in India can usually be arranged for $10,000–$12,000.

India, Israel, and Georgia allow surrogacy although Russia requires a medical reason for it, but some countries like Canada, Japan, the People's Republic of China, and Saudi Arabia do not permit it at all. Thailand and Ukraine are other popular sources for an international clientele, while Nepal and Poland are quickly gaining in reputations.

In an article by Marcia C. Inhorn in November 2015, the European Society for Human Reproduction and Embryology (ESHRE) Taskforce on Cross Border Reproductive Care published the results of a large study involving 46 IVF clinics in six European destinations (Belgium, the Czech Republic, Denmark, Slovenia, Spain, and Switzerland). Based on 1,230 patient questionnaires, the study estimated a minimum of 20,000–30,000 cross-border IVF cycles each year involving 11,000–14,000 patients.

According to *Yale News* (October 2015), reproductive travel is not only fueled by monetary savings but also by such factors as resource shortages; legal, religious, and ethical obstacles; quality of care; and cultural issues related to privacy and social comfort. For instance, a service where a couple lives may be lacking because it is not considered safe enough or some individuals may not be able to receive a service at public expense due to age, marital status, or sexual orientation. Thus, they may turn to reproductive tourism.

Still, expenses are the strongest reason for seeking reproductive tourism. For instance, although most Africans do not have access to IVF technology, wealthier Africans—usually from countries like Sudan, Ethiopia, or Somalia—have the monetary means to travel to reproductive destinations like Dubai. In her book *Cosmopolitan Conceptions: IVF Sojourns in Global Dubai* (Duke University Press, 2015) Yale professor Marcia C. Inhorn defines "repro-travelers" to Dubai as people who wish to evade laws and receive high-quality safe care. Inhorn interviewed couples from 50 different countries, including India, Pakistan, the United States, and Australia, who used the fertility clinic Conceive in Dubai. Couples from the Middle East liked traveling to a society that understood their strong cultural mandate to have children and the Islamic religion's stigmatization of infertility and ban on adoption.

A 2010 global survey listed between 4,000 and 4,500 IVF clinics, with more than one-quarter located in Japan and India. Other nations with large numbers of IVF clinics include the United States (450–480); Italy (360); Spain (177–203); Korea (142); Germany (120–121); and China (102–300), according to Marcia C. Inhorn and Pasquale Patrizio in *Human Reproduction Update* (March 2015).

Another reason couples travel outside their home territory is for access to PGD, which has been available since 1994 and tests embryos for genetic traits that predispose them to severe diseases like cystic fibrosis and sickle cell anemia. Some countries allow PGD; others limit the practice, and still others (Algeria, Austria, Chile, China, Ireland, the Ivory Coast, and the Philippines) prohibit it.

Mexico

Although IVF in the United States can cost between $18,000 and $20,000, the same treatment in Mexico runs from $3,500 to $5,000. Even taking into account the cost of travel—including lodging, food, and medicines—the tourism alternative ends up being cheaper. For that reason, Mexico is marketed by some fertility concierges as a resort where women can combine the discomfort of ART with pleasant scenery and a temperate climate.

Czech Republic

A similar approach is taken in the Czech Republic. A company called IVF Holiday advertises on the Internet, stating that an infertility trip abroad can lower stress levels and promote conception. Whether it does or not is debatable, but author Amy Speier, a medical anthropologist at the University of Texas, documents the journeys of 29 American tourists to Czech clinics in her book *Fertility Holidays: IVF Tourism and the Reproduction of Whiteness* (NYU Press, 2016). She says people in need of IVF go there because the price is lower than in the United States and the legislation is liberal (regulations stipulate only that sperm and egg donations should be voluntary, anonymous, and compensated at approximately 1,000 euros). The fee for an egg donor costs North Americans only $4,000. Compare that with the $25,000–$40,000 for a round of IVF American women often pay. Even with travel expenses, the IVF price is far less.

Turkey

Turkey is another heavily trafficked destination. Ranked seventh in the global IVF market and with more than 120 assisted reproduction centers (according to a 2016 paper in *BMC Health Services Research*), Turkey has made IVF accessible through state subsidization and funding of two IVF cycles for all Turkish citizens of all socioeconomic backgrounds. The cost of medical services is only about 30–50 percent of the costs in

Western Europe and the United States, and the success rate in Turkey is better than in the United States. On the other hand, Turkey's volatile political climate could potentially shut down medical tourism there.

India and Ukraine

India also profits nicely since according to a 2015 paper in *Risk Management and Healthcare Policy*, India lifted its ban on surrogacy in 2002. Its 3,000 specialty clinics take in approximately $400 million annually. In Ukraine surrogacy births have increased by 20 percent a year and could rise to 40 percent by 2020 with the opening of several large clinics. Married couples from abroad make up about 50 percent of the total number of Ukraine's surrogacy cycles. Lenient surrogacy laws as well as comparatively low prices attract clients. Surrogacy in the United States may cost up to $100,000, but in Ukraine, the price can be three to four times cheaper, according to *Suffolk Transnational Law Review* (September 2013).

Reproductive Tourism Disadvantages

While cost is the number one reason for reproductive tourism's use, disadvantages also exist: the risk of infectious, communicable diseases or genetic disorders; language barriers; emotional challenges; and an inexpensive-on-paper price with additional "surprise" costs tacked on.

The worst problems are legal ones, which may affect citizenship status for the child, marital status, and sexual orientation. Another complication is transporting frozen embryos from a clinic in the United States to an international clinic. Also, some countries like Italy, Austria, Norway, Sweden, and Switzerland ban egg donations completely; others have banned compensation for egg donations.

To avoid ART disasters, couples need to check that the foreign clinic they are using addresses the same health factors as SART does. Also, the use of concierge services can ease the way but must be checked out carefully to avoid a potential disaster as in the case of Planet Hospital, a Los Angeles-based service that ultimately filed for bankruptcy with clients losing thousands of dollars. (For more information on repro tourism, contact the surrogacy and egg donation agency Family Inceptions International in Georgia, familyinceptions.com).

ALTERNATIVE TREATMENTS

Before undertaking invasive ART procedures in the United States or abroad, couples can invest in some alternative treatments or, at the very least, combine them with ART to help women feel more comfortable and in control while undergoing IVF. According to a new study from the University of Louisville, Kentucky, women's high stress levels reduce their probability of conception by up to 45 percent. Other experts, however, deny a correlation between stress and fertility. Obviously the jury is still out on this point.

Some stress-relieving procedures include herbs, yoga, biofeedback, aerobic exercise, guided imagery, journaling, music therapy, meditation, mind-body methods, mindfulness, progressive muscle relaxation, cognitive behavioral therapy, and visualization.

Here are other fertility techniques:

Massage Therapy

Massage therapy, often referred to as Mayan Abdominal Massage, applies a holistic approach and is best for repositioning incorrectly functioning uteruses as well as for adhesions caused by procedures like fibroid removal, endometriosis, and cesarean delivery.

Sleep

Yes, sleep. Sleep can affect male ART. A study headed by a Boston University epidemiologist followed 790 couples (October 19, 2016). Researchers examined both short and long sleep durations and found that men who slept less than six or more than nine hours a night had a 42 percent reduced probability of conception in any given month. The reason is hormonal, researchers concluded. Fertility experts know that testosterone is crucial for reproduction, and the majority of daily testosterone release in men occurs during sleep.

Hypnotherapy

Hypnotherapy's success rate is based on its ability to relieve underlying anxiety and stress. The hypnotherapist plants a positive suggestion in a person's mind while the person is under hypnosis. The therapist emphasizes a statement or some kind of mantra aimed at making a person feel calmer or more confident. The person can recall it later to manage his or her own stress levels.

In one study published by the ESHRE, the success rates of IVF doubled in women who underwent ART and hypnotherapy at the same time. Conducted by a team at Soroka Hospital in Beersheva, Israel, this study of 185 women found that 28 percent of the IVF patients who were hypnotized became pregnant compared to 14 percent of the control group. Eliahu Levitas, who headed the investigation, indicated that tranquilizers had been used in prior studies, but nothing works as well as hypnosis. Also, Dr. Shobha Gupta, of India, uses hypnotherapy and meditation to relax overwrought clients and claims that the process improves the conception rates during IVF cycles. She has used hypnosis on 206 women so far, and about 65 percent of them conceived.

Mind-Body

Psychologist Alice Domar, director of the Boston-based Mind-Body Center for Women IVF, suggests that mind-body techniques can elicit a relaxation response that reduces stress and increases a couple's chances of conception.

Weight and Supplements

Weight management has a profound effect on fertility. Being over- or underweight disrupts the hormonal balance and can cause menstrual irregularities and prevent ovulation. Studies also indicate that obesity can negatively impact embryo quality even in younger women under age 35 who are undergoing IVF.

Supplementation also can aid in conception. For women desiring maximum fertility, the recommended dose of folic acid is 400 micrograms per day. Vitamin D supplementation may be associated with higher fertilization rates, according to a September 2016 study in *American Journal of Clinical Nutrition*. Unfortunately, higher fertilization rates do not translate to a higher pregnancy or live birth rate. On the other hand, in a 2013 *Cochrane Review* article, when men took antioxidants like melatonin, zinc, and vitamins C, A, and E, the result was significantly higher live birth rates in ART. Women did not get the same response. However, according to Laura Berman, assistant professor of obstetrics/gynecology and psychiatry at Northwestern University, a 2018 NIH (National Institutes of Health) study suggests that women low in iodine have half the chance of conceiving as women who have healthy levels of iodine.

Chiropractic

According to the American Pregnancy Association (May 2017), chiropractic care can supplement other fertility treatments due to its high safety record. It can benefit women with fertility issues associated with improper nervous system function, poor nutrition, high stress, and negative lifestyle habits since chiropractors reduce interference in the nervous system. Best of all, chiropractic care is cost effective. It can help patients avoid IVF entirely or reduce the number of IVF cycles needed to achieve conception.

Acupuncture

Acupuncture's effectiveness in reducing stress, balancing hormones, and improving blood flow to the reproductive organs is well recognized although a 2013 review in *Human Reproduction Update* found no overall benefit. On the other hand, according to the ASRM, acupuncture is recommended for polycystic ovary syndrome, fibroids, endometriosis, ovarian reserve, and sperm quality issues. Acupuncture also may help relieve side effects from fertility drugs such as bloating and nausea. Women are advised to start acupuncture three months before they begin IVF or intrauterine device (IUD). The National Certification Commission for Acupuncture and Oriental Medicine and the American Board of Medical Acupuncture can supply names of competent practitioners. (See resources at end of book.)

THE ADOPTION OPTION

Not all couples want to face the financial, medical, emotional, and logistical challenges inherent in IVF, IUD, or surrogacy. Even alternative treatments can bother some people. Sometimes adoption can seem like the best choice. According to the website Reproductivefacts.org, adoption decisions often result from a distaste for fertility treatments while other couples adopt only after fertility treatments fail.

History of Adoption

According to Debora L. Spar in *The Baby Business*, adoption goes back to Grecian times when childless couples often adopted heirs. In Rome, couples with biological children frequently adopted, sometimes selecting more attractive children to displace their own genetic offspring. The underlying motivation was economic. Parents felt they needed the right kind of descendant to protect their fortunes and preserve their family name. During the Middle Ages, families did not adopt as their predecessors had. Despite the reality of families possessing distinct bloodlines, they would "take in" children from unrelated families. These children might serve as apprentices or servants, remaining in these positions until they reached the age when common law would consider them independent.

As early as 1627 in America, 1,400 poor or orphaned children were apprenticed directly to the Virginia Company. Economic necessity dictated the need for more workers. In 1740, one wealthy Georgia planter took in 61 orphans to join his family and work in the fields. By the mid-nineteenth century, financial necessity had started to transition from worker-slave status to informal family ties. Adoption cases began emerging in state courts, usually involving issues of contested inheritance. In 1858, for instance, the nieces and nephews of a then-recently deceased Louisiana man sued to inherit his property. The relatives argued that his adopted daughter had no legal rights to his estate. The state court disagreed, however, and ruled in favor of the adopted daughter. Litigation like this ensued in various regions of the country, so state legislatures began enacting explicit legislation to give adopted children the right of inheritance. The result was an increase in adoption.

Around this same time, however, the children of immigrants began flooding urban areas like Boston, New York, and Chicago, overwhelming the public houses that took them in. Social reformers intervened and began to construct private children's agencies and philanthropic institutions to care for orphaned or abandoned children. The most well-known of these organizations was the Children's Aid Society of New York, which was founded in 1853 by a Protestant minister, who later set up a program of orphan trains that shipped children to farm families in the Midwest. The status of these children was a mix of adoption and servitude, but this endeavor showed that adoption by strangers could work. Other religious agencies copied the Children's Aid Society model and assigned children to homes in the Midwest.

Over time upper-class women began "saving" babies born to unwed mothers, delivering them to friends or acquaintances looking for a child. Other baby brokers sprang up: hospital nurses, private maternity homes, and local court officials. Between 1920 and 1935 most of the country's largest child service organizations began to offer and promote adoption, employing social workers and applying to certain agencies for licenses. Over the next several decades, adoption became more regulated by the U.S. Children's Bureau. As a result, independent adoption agencies soon began competing with the state-licensed ones. Estimates by the Children's Bureau suggest that about half of American adoptions in the 1940s occurred outside the domain of licensed adoption agencies.

When licensed agencies began handling illegitimate births in the aftermath of World War II, adoptions increased significantly because the agencies became more open-minded about placing children across religious and racial lines. Between 1938 and 1965 the number of adoptions in the United States soared from 16,000 a year to 142,000. In 1955, the U.S. Congress investigated the illicit baby trade and found evidence of an interstate market that generated as much as $15 million a year. Between 1946 and 1970 more than 2 million children were adopted through a combination of licensed agencies and independent providers.

Adoption Today

Today, adoptions can be arranged through a private, county, or state agency or can be organized independently—either internationally or domestically. Independent adoptions usually involve doctors, counselors, facilitators, and attorneys. Adoption laws differ from state to state and country to country, and expenses as well as wait times vary widely. Many domestic adoptions are open adoptions where the birth parents and adoptive parents share information. This differs from international adoptions where little information about the child or birth parents is available.

RESOLVE, the national infertility association established in 1974, not only supports ART but also favors adoption. For example, its Gift of Adoption Fund gives grants ranging from $1,000 to $7,500 with an average amount of $3,500. A Child Waits Foundation provides low-interest loans up to $10,000 to help defray the costs of an international adoption as well as grants under $5,000. Grants are also available through grants.gov—the Children's Bureau and the U.S. Department of Health and Human Services. Adoptive parents may also qualify for a federal tax credit up to $12,150.

Materials on the aforementioned sites can help prospective parents choose the best adoption route for them. For example, if the couple wishes to use an agency, RESOLVE has a checklist of criteria that includes a list of complaints filed against the State Department of Social Services, what healthy children are available, what the agency's position is on open adoption, what foreign countries or orphanages the agency works with, what medical information is available, what kind of contract is required between the birth parents and the prospective adoptive parents, and what the average age of the child is at placement and arrival.

RESOLVE also has caveats: Watch out if the agency asks for a large amount of money beyond the retainer and before the birth parent is located. Also, proceed with caution if there is little information about the birth parents' ethnic, medical, educational, and social backgrounds or if no one from the agency or lawyer's office is present at the first meeting of the birth parents and the prospective adoptive parents. RESOLVE supplies resources and links to organizations such as the North American Council on Adoptable Children, the Joint Council of International Children's Services, and the Center for Adoption Support and Education, Inc.

In a typical domestic adoption, the prospective parents pay a preliminary fee—usually between $100 and $500—to the agency; then they pay between $700 and $3,000 for a home study to determine the suitability of the prospective parents. If a child is found for the couple, the parents then pay a placement fee, which varies from $6,500 to more than $50,000.

Parents also generally cover the birth mother's medical expenses and costs of living during the pregnancy, according to *The Baby Business* by Debora L. Spar. The author also says U.S. families adopt more than 100,000 children each year—about 15 percent from abroad and nearly all through state-sanctioned channels such as Children's Home and Aid Society of Illinois, Christian Child Placement Services, and Jewish Family Services. As of 2004, the average costs of an infant adoption in the United States ranged between $10,000 and $40,000, but in a handful of cases, prices ran as high as $100,000.

Many couples also work with adoption attorneys or independent brokers who link the couple directly with birth parents. Most brokers charge an hourly rate of $200–$350. Prices for international adoptions in Russia, Guatemala, China, India, and Ethiopia vary. A white Russian child might cost about $15,000, while a black child from Ethiopia can go from $6,700 to $8,000. Children of other ethnicities fall somewhere in the middle range—from a Filipino child ($6,000) to a Chinese child ($7,000) to a Colombian child ($8,900). Handicapped children are frequently offered with a scholarship or financial assistance. Foreign adoption agencies include Families Thru International Adoption, Commonwealth Adoptions, MAPS International, Angels' Haven, Holt International, and Wide Horizons for Children.

Conclusion

This chapter presented alternatives to traditional ART. It summarized some of the alternative treatments to infertility such as acupuncture and chiropractic as well as another infertility pathway: adoption. Another option to contracting for ART services in the United States is reproductive tourism, and several countries are cited as areas where medical tourism has established itself as a profitable industry and alternate venue for IVF or surrogacy.

PGD also is an option that has great appeal for some people—usually those concerned about an embryonic child carrying the gene for an undesirable disease such as Tay Sachs. For these people, PGD is worthwhile, even given the fact that the woman must first consent to IVF in order to scan her embryos for problems.

Next in Chapter 3 is a discussion of the pricing scales of various ART procedures in the United States and how the lack of governmental regulations has created a dearth of health policies in the insurance market to the point that only 15 states provide any coverage at all for infertility.

Financing Fertility

Kristina D. and her husband Brian tried to get pregnant naturally for a year. Then in 2014 they visited a fertility clinic and opted for three trials of artificial insemination (AI), which failed. The couple then tried in vitro fertilization (IVF), and finally—after about $18,000 out-of-pocket expenses for IVF and chromosomal testing (including $3,000 for 60–70 doctors' visits and co-pays)—Kristina became pregnant. Her husband's employer—their sole beneficiary for health care—did not cover Kristina's fertility treatments or drugs, so the entire financial responsibility fell on the couple.

This is the usual scenario for most Assisted Reproductive Technology (ART) patients because of the United States' unregulated policies on infertility procedures and its neglect of health insurance mandates. This unfortunate reality makes the United States an outlier compared to the rest of the developed world.

As previously noted, ART prices are staggering, and in general, average U.S. costs are much more than average global costs. This chapter focuses on the expense range for different fertility procedures, legal and other costs, the price of egg and sperm donations, insurance coverage and/or employment benefits (among civilians and veterans), out-of-pocket costs, and the 15 states with mandated insurance requirements.

THE ART MARKET

According to author Debora L. Spar's chart on "The U.S. Market for Fertility Treatment, 2004" (*The Baby Business*), the total cost for fertility treatments in the United States in 2004 was nearly $3 billion for the million-plus Americans who underwent fertility protocols. In 2015 investment banking company Harris Williams and Co. estimated U.S. costs rose to between $3 and $4 billion. ART services also include the handling of eggs and sperm, which are estimated to cost $1.7–$2.5 billion. Demand for fertility services in the United States is forecasted to grow approximately 4 percent for the next several years due to such factors as aging, increasing obesity, and cultural shifts.

In 2015 the 33 European Union countries pushed the global ART market to $22.3 billion, and a new report by the business consulting firm Grand View Research predicted that the market will increase to 29.3 billion by 2022. Frozen nondonor gametes are identified as the most lucrative segment of ART growth. Harris Williams predicts an even healthier global market of $30–$40 billion, the largest consumers being Europe, Japan, Australia, and Brazil.

Costs of Gametes

Eggs and sperm are the basic building blocks for fertilization, and their costs can vary. For instance, according to *The Baby Business* by Debora L. Spar, the cost of eggs can range anywhere from $4,500 to $50,000, but the American Society for Reproductive Medicine (ASRM) recommends payments of $5,000–$10,000. Sperm are more plentiful and easier to procure, and this is reflected in their lower prices, which usually range from $50 to $200 plus a fee for the sperm bank or brokerage agency.

According to *The Baby Business*, many gametes are priced at $300 for sperm and $4,500 for eggs. The controversial egg market surfaced in the early 1990s. At first eggs came mainly from the intended recipient's friends and family or possibly a college roommate, but as infertility procedures became more popular, altruistic donors became scarcer. Fertility clinics began cropping up, going commercial and advertising for egg donors. Offering a fee of about $2,500, clinics posted notices on college campuses for healthy women willing to help infertile couples for a fee.

Eventually commercialism expanded. For example, Shelley Smith, a family counselor in Beverly Hills, California, placed ads in 1991 in publications geared to young actresses, handpicking them for attractiveness, intelligence, good health, and psychological balance. Catering to an upscale clientele, Smith's Center for Egg Donation charged her clients $4,500. Competition emerged from other players such as Bill Handel's Center for Surrogate Parenting and the Virginia-based Genetics & IVF Institute as well as many small-time brokers. Soon egg prices increased and ranged between $3,000 and $8,000—for instance, those in Washington, D.C., averaged about $5,000 and those in New York at $7,500–$8,000.

For the right amount of cash, clients could sometimes learn more than just the physical and social facts of their prospective donors. At the Genetics & IVF Institute and other elite agencies, clients learned their donor's ethnic background, SAT scores, college-level athletic ability, education record, occupation, musical preferences, and special interests. Some businesses catered to niche buyers—for instance, Asian couples or homosexuals. And because commercial donation remains illegal in most industrialized countries other than the United States, U.S. gamete firms cash in. For example, at the Center for Egg Donation in Colorado, 30 percent of its business in 2003 came from abroad, with the numbers of foreign clients steadily rising. Harris William says the typical one-time cost for donor eggs is $15,000–$20,000.

Commercial sperm banks have been around since 1970—longer than egg marketers. The first for-profit sperm bank opened in Minnesota. Many women wanted sperm since their partners either had genetic diseases or were impotent or sterile. Some women had no husband but still desired children. As with egg banks, patients initially used sperm only from known persons such as their husbands, friends, or family. Then, by 1980, 17 frozen-sperm banks had popped up across the United States, furnishing raw material for 20,000 babies at about $66 per specimen.

Donors were hired through promotional materials, and specialty companies appeared. For example, the Repository for Germinal Choice in Escondido, California, which operated between 1980 and 1999, offered only the sperm of Nobel Prize winners, Olympic athletes, and other exceptional persons. Other enterprises catered to lesbian couples. In 1988, the U.S. government surveyed the AI market and found that 22 percent of AI users employed commercially purchased semen.

For the standard $200–$300 fee, sperm banks reveal a set list of their donors' characteristics. For example, California Cryobank in Los Angeles, California, provides more than 20 pages of information, including religion, hair texture, occupation, and education. After the semen is collected, the sperm is washed, flash frozen, and suspended in a tank of liquid nitrogen. (Under federal regulation, all sperm must be kept in storage for at least six months while the donor is repeatedly tested for HIV, hepatitis, and sexually transmitted diseases [STDs].)

In 2000 the *Wall Street Journal* estimated the global market for sperm to be between $50 million and $100 million a year. The amounts are high due to a 2,000 percent markup. Donors receive around $75 per specimen, and each specimen yields between three and six vials of sperm, each vial selling for $250–$400. According to market research company Grand View Research, the global male infertility market size was estimated at $3.1 billion in 2016. Increasing infertility rates and the spread of ART are expected to be key factors driving the global market growth.

ESTIMATED EXPENSES FOR SURROGACY

Men Having Babies, Inc. (MHB), a New York City-based nonprofit organization serving gays, helps their clients manage surrogacy and egg donation purchases. In 2015 the agency put together two charts—one pertaining to surrogacy and the other to egg donation (*ABA Guide to Assisted Reproduction*, ABA, 2016). To arrive at cost estimates of surrogacy and egg donation, people need to add up the totals of both tables, which cite such costs as donor matching, legal fees, medical screening, and other nonmedical and medical expenses. According to the *ABA Guide to Assisted Reproduction*, these totals would amount to a minimum of $83,000 for surrogacy and a likely cost of $122,000. The typical cost for the high end of the spectrum is $191,000. Harris Williams approximates the typical cost of surrogacy at $50,000–$100,000.

Stem Cell–Derived Gametes

Stem cell research in the United States will continue to compete with other countries like China, Korea, and the United Kingdom. Since 2000 the overall U.S. federal research funding for stem cell research is several billion dollars. People who cannot produce healthy gametes but who want to have "children of their own" will drive continued research.

According to Greely, about 20,000 women and 5,000 men would be interested in replacing donor gametes with those derived from their own stem cells. Additionally, over 30,000 women in the United States age 40 and over would also be interested in their own stem cell–derived eggs. The fact that the age of motherhood continues to rise may encourage a powerful market for stem cell–derived gametes. Consider this: If 50,000 people a year who are infertile due to gamete problems paid just $1,000 for a stem cell–derived gamete, that would produce an anticipated market of $50 million per year in the United States alone. And this is not counting the LGBT population of 200,000 to 1 million couples who also might want stem cell gametes. Thus, a heavy demand already exists, and like contraception and IVF, the medical and entrepreneurial markets will probably respond accordingly.

COSTS OF MULTIPLES

In a study at the ASRM 2015 annual meeting, a team of Boston investigators examined the hospital costs of singletons (single births) versus triplet births. Singletons saved hospitals over $4 billion. Triplet pregnancies were estimated to be 11–27 times more expensive than singletons. A 2014 Netherlands study in *Human Reproduction* showed that the risk of hospitalization for outpatient visits and medical procedures was higher for multiples. The reason for this is that children in multiple pregnancies suffer poorer neonatal outcomes such as preterm birth, complications, underweight births, and low birth rate. They also require more medical care immediately and later in life (2005 Centers for Disease Control and Prevention [CDC] Report). Fertility doctors are heeding these financial figures and are beginning to transfer fewer embryos. In 2016 the CDC reported that the number and rate of triplet and higher-order multiple births in the United States fell 41 percent between 1998 and 2014.

Transferring three or more embryos is more common in states without an insurance mandate because women are forced to limit the number of cycles. As a result, they increase their odds of conception by implanting multiple embryos. In states with an insurance mandate, women implanted fewer embryos, says the CDC in April 2016. These improvements in transfers, however, had more to do with overall improvements in ART practices rather than in insurance mandates.

Consider, for instance, the case of Teresa Anderson. In 2005 she agreed to be a gestational surrogate for $15,000. To increase the chance of pregnancy, doctors transplanted five embryos into Anderson. They all survived, and although the public relations effect for the doctor and hospital was great, these babies were extraordinarily expensive—more than $400,000.

SURROGACY AND SINGLETON COSTS

Reduction in multiple embryo transfer reduces the adverse economic impact of surrogate pregnancy. The ASRM-SART guidelines have been revised to reduce the number of transferred embryos, and this recommendation has already eliminated over 13,000 high-order multiple pregnancies and saved the U.S. government more than $4 billion. Objections to the singleton mind-set have surfaced, however, because it limits individual choice and autonomy—ethical concepts often cited for their mass appeal.

States also vary in surrogacy costs because some prohibit the use of the term "compensation." They prefer altruistic surrogacy in which the surrogate does not get a fee but rather the prospective parents pay the surrogate's out-of-pocket and medical expenses. Other expense categories, however, can further increase the bill: life insurance, a disability policy for the surrogate, payments for start of medication, mock cycles (to prepare the body for the real embryo transfer), embryo transfers, monthly allowances, maternity clothes, and surrogates' travel costs.

According to the *ABA Guide to Assisted Reproduction Techniques*, other costs also can include payments for loss of reproductive organs, embryo transfer cancellation fees, selective reduction or elective terminations, invasive procedures that require overnight hospital stays or administration of IV fluids, ectopic pregnancies (a pregnancy in which the fetus develops outside the uterus, typically in a fallopian tube), miscarriages, cesarean sections, multiple births, bed rest ordered by the physician, childcare, housekeeping, and breast milk pumping.

POTENTIAL LEGAL COSTS

Legal expenses mainly refer to the surrogacy situation, which, as already explained, can vary in the United States from state to state and depend on the couple's unique situation. Because the ART world is unregulated, intended parents must pay for all costs such as legal representation (average bills are $6,000–$12,000). For that fee, the attorney drafts, negotiates, and reviews the surrogacy contract for the intended parents, ensuring that the intended parents are named as the legal parents on the birth certificate and administering monies between the two parties. The intended parents' attorney also drafts, reviews, obtains signatures, and files legal pleading papers with the court. The exact filing costs are determined by the state where the baby is to be born and range from $500 to $3,000. An escrow account is also held by the attorney or a bonded third party to guarantee the surrogate's reimbursement.

Legal costs also can relate to a donated egg or sperm, embryo donation, or embryo adoption. The two main legal concerns relating to genetic donation are ensuring that the donor of the genetic material is not deemed a legal parent and that the intended parents are in possession of the donated genetic material after it is frozen and if the parties separate, divorce, or die. To avoid possible disputes, it is recommended that the intended parents offer legal representation by an ART attorney to the genetic donors. This expense, of course, is necessarily absorbed by the intended parents, and fees for these services vary throughout the United States.

Costs of SET (Single Embryo Transplant)

According to *Contraception and Reproductive Medicine* (2016), the new gold standard for IVF is a singleton—an elective single embryo transfer or eSET. This new standard is due to scientific advances in embryo cryopreservation, blastocyst selection, and preimplantation genetic diagnosis (PGD). The higher costs of IVF complications from multiple embryos explain why SET is the mandated fertility coverage in Europe, Canada, and selected states in the United States.

The ASRM reported in 2015 that singleton gestations cost between $17,000 and $24,000 for pregnancy, delivery, and up to one year of neonatal care—much less than multiples. Furthermore, a study comparing the cost effectiveness of intrauterine insemination (IUI) with IVF with SETs showed that IVF strategies were found to be more expensive without being more effective (Tjon-Kon-Fat et al., *Human Reproduction*, 2015). Harris Williams says typical costs for IVF are $12,000 compared to $1,000–$2,000 for IUI.

In 2015 the ASRM conducted a survey of 235 patients and found that patients preferred to carry and deliver one child at a time. In 2012 the ASRM reported that when IVF was paid by insurance or risk-sharing programs, more patients preferred eSET.

Published studies of cost-effectiveness of eSET show similar costs for eSET and double embryo transplant (DET), but the results of a Netherlands study suggest that after patient education, patients change their preferences to eSET. According to a 2014 study published in *Reproductive BioMedicine Online*, the national savings from fewer multiple births would be over $6 billion a year in the United States.

SMART COST-SAVING

Despite the staggering costs for ART, couples can do several things to minimize their cash flow. For instance, women who plan to delay child-bearing until age 40 can save money if they have their eggs harvested before age 38 (Mesen et al., *Fertility and Sterility*, June 2015). Also, cutting out unnecessary drugs ($3,000–$5,000 per IVF cycle), tests, or procedures can simplify methods and save money. Furthermore, lower doses of pricey IVF drugs can be used for mild IVF approaches—a protocol increasingly popular in countries like Japan, France, and the Netherlands. Intracytoplasmic sperm injection (ICSI; sperm inserted directly into the egg in cases of male infertility) also can be eliminated for many couples since faulty sperm affects only 40 percent of infertile couples (in 2010 it was used in nearly 70 percent of IVF cycles globally). ICSI, which adds $1,500 to the cost, is more expensive than IVF alone and can be dispensed with if the male sperm is normal.

IVF Lab in a Box

An ART procedure that resembles a shoebox-sized IVF lab also may eventually prove to be a cost saver, according to the *Economist* (August 2016). The gametes are placed in a cheap glass tube connected to another tube in which the carbon dioxide needed for fertilization is produced using baking soda. So far 51 babies have been born this way in Belgium with success rates comparable to those for conventional IVF. In Europe this method cuts IVF costs by three-quarters, says Willem Ombelet of the Genk Institute for Fertility Technology in Belgium. The temperature-controlled technique boosts the woman's odds of pregnancy by more than a quarter, and the stable environment gives the embryos a better chance of implantation in the uterus. Also, smart blastocyst selections after fertilization and a PGD add-on can help to ensure the transfer of healthy elective single embryos without compromising outcomes.

The INVOcell Device

Approved by Health Canada in 2015, the INVOcell device may one day cut the price of IVF in half. On the company's website (invobioscience .com), it advertises the product's use in 11 states (including New York, Arizona, and California), Calgary, Canada, Colombia, Brazil, India, and parts of Europe. To keep costs down, fertility doctor Kevin Doody, codirector of the Center for Assisted Reproduction in Bedford, Texas, prescribes fertility drugs conservatively, basing the amount on body weight and anti-Mullerian hormone testing (which estimates egg supply). He allows the gametes to mingle for an hour or so with sperm and then places the as-yet-unfertilized eggs with sperm clinging to the outer shells into the INVOcell. This device is inserted inside the woman's vagina, secured by a diaphragm, and left there for five days. When Dr. Doody conducted a trial of 40 women (half receiving traditional IVF and half receiving the INVO-cell), the rates of fertilization, pregnancy, and live birth were similar in both groups (*Canadian Medical Association Journal*, February 2015). In a Food and Drug Administration (FDA) study of INVOcell, just over half of patients conceived in one cycle, and some had leftover embryos to freeze for future use. The cost of INVOcell is slightly greater than the cost of three cycles of IUI and approximately half of the cost of traditional IVF, so some couples may elect to skip IUI and proceed directly to INVOcell.

Refund Programs

In a study in the *International Journal of Fertility and Sterility* (Jafarzadeh-Kenarsari et al., April–June 2015), American patients some-times sold their houses or took out home equity loans to pay for infertility treatments. To ease costs, many clinics now offer success or refund pro-grams for six cycles. If a woman does not get pregnant, she may get her money back. Some doctors feel that there are major ethical issues to this arrangement since the program is only made available to patients likely to become pregnant in the first few cycles. Other clinics offer discounts to patients who opt for SETs. By offering incentives for certain treatment options, these programs can influence patient decisions based on financial rather than medically scientific reasons.

Funds for Fertility

Without health insurance or incentive programs, couples may tap into savings, overcharge credit cards, and plead for cash from parents and fam-ilies. Other couples take out loans from fertility-finance companies, some-times at high interest rates. For instance, IntegraMed Fertility, a network of American fertility clinics, helps couples get loans from fertility-finance firms.

Also, many fertility nonprofits offer help. The Tinina Q Cade Founda-tion holds fund-raisers for opportunities to receive free IVF cycles and donates as much as $10,000 to infertility patients. Other grant-giving organizations are the Baby Quest Foundation, which provides $2,000–$16,000 grants, and Savannah Grove ($10,000). The Pay It Forward Fer-tility Foundation helps as do the International Council on Infertility Infor-mation Dissemination, the JFCS Fertility Fund, and the Kevin J. Lederer Foundation, which awards $10,000 Kevin J. Lederer Life Foundation grants.

Adoption organizations also give grants. The National Adoption Foundation Financial Programs awards grants to adoptive parents four times a year. Other similar organizations include the Gift of Adoption Fund whose grants range from $2,000 to $5,000 for adopting children with serious medical issues and for low-income families. Help Us Adopt.ORG awards grants of up to $15,000.

Getting the Most from a Fertility Clinic

Fertility clinics in the United States are not all created equal, especially in pricing. Asking the right questions can help couples choose top-rated clinics with fair fees and good success rates. RESOLVE: The National Fertility Organization recommends vetting fertility clinics regarding payment and advising patients on physician costs. Patients should weigh factors like staff expertise, reputation, and location. If cost predominates as a factor, patients need to ask the clinic for a detailed list of procedures and corresponding costs.

Other suggested questions:

Are medications, tests, lab work, ultrasounds, and consultations included?
What are the costs (including screening) when using an egg donor, sperm donor, or surrogate?
What are the average costs associated with medications?
Does medical insurance cover any of the medications, testing, monitoring, or procedures?
Does the fertility clinic have a detailed list of procedures and costs for such specific procedures as IVF, IUI, ICSI, and PGD as well as storage fees for frozen embryos?
Does the clinic offer a reduced rate if the patient purchases an IVF package?

Endometrial Surgery Costs

Another cost savings might be to reconsider having endometrial surgery as a cure for fertility. In Salt Lake City, Utah, at a 2016 ASRM meeting, data analysts examined the insurance costs faced by women with endometriosis according to types of treatment. For instance, surgical patients faced higher costs than nonsurgical patients, who could opt for laparoscopy or laparotomy. Surgical patients had higher costs due partially to indirect costs such as short-term disability payments and absence from work. The website ReproductiveFacts.org says surgery can exceed $34,000.

According to ASRM, physicians always knew women faced physical and emotional difficulties with endometrial treatment, but the data now also show a high financial cost. Furthermore, ASRM determined that the research on the treatment of endometriosis to eliminate infertility shows that few infertile women undergoing laparoscopy become pregnant.

In short, the smart move may be to skip the endometrial laparoscopy and opt for an ART procedure.

U.S. ART Insurance

The annual ART growth rate of the United States is 5 percent compared to Europe's rate of 7.5 percent and Australia's 9 percent. American physician-scientists at Brown University attribute the lesser rate in the United States to high under- and uninsurance rates, high out-of-pocket expenditures for public payers, and reluctant private payers. As a result, most people in the United States with health insurance do not have infertility coverage.

If they do have coverage, policy limitations in the 15 states that offer it can minimize payouts, according to the website Attainivf.attainfertility .com. For example, some states do not cover the use of donor sperm or egg or only include certain types of infertility treatments. Coverage also can determine who performs the treatment and where it is performed, stipulate limits on how many IVF cycles will be covered, mandate age cut-offs, or be capped at a certain amount.

Since the 1980s 13 states have laws that require insurance companies to cover infertility treatment. Louisiana and New York prohibit the exclusion of coverage for a medical problem resulting in infertility, and two states—California and Texas—have laws requiring insurance companies to offer coverage for infertility treatment. Utah requires insurers that provide coverage for maternity benefits to provide an indemnity benefit for adoption or infertility treatments. Unfortunately, California, Louisiana, and New York have laws that specifically exclude coverage for IVF.

Mandatory coverage has not yet been mainstreamed in the United States, possibly because there is no standard coverage for expenses incurred in typical adoptions or conceptions. Expenses run from one extreme to the other. Costs for adoptions or conceptions differ dramatically from clinic to clinic and from state to state. Standardization might force society to decide whether ART is a luxury or a medical necessity.

The irony of this price war is that a 2003 Harris Interactive Inc. Survey revealed that 80 percent of the general population felt that infertility treatments should be covered by insurance. However, according to Harvard professor Deborah Spar's estimates, only a little more than one-third of the infertile seek fertility treatments. One reason is the population most likely to be concerned about fertility treatment is also the least likely to have health insurance—those between the ages of 18 and 35. Most states with insurance laws guarantee fertility coverage for IVF, but public programs like Medicaid treat fertility issues as elective procedures and remain uncovered.

RESOLVE: The National Fertility Organization endorses state and federal legislation that requires insurers to cover the costs of appropriate medical treatment. In 2010 the organization lobbied to have fertility treatments included as one of the basic health benefits under the Affordable Care Act, but contraception and maternity care made the cut, not infertility treatments.

MASSACHUSETTS: A MODEL INSURANCE PROGRAM

Massachusetts was the first state to enact an infertility mandate. According to a 2006 employer survey commissioned by RESOLVE, 91 percent of Massachusetts residents and others offered infertility treatments have not experienced an increase in their medical costs because of this coverage. Furthermore, in a 1998 study in *Fertility and Sterility* the cost of infertility services as a percent of the total health premiums decreased after the 1987 Massachusetts mandate for state-covered universal health insurance.

Massachusetts transplants Margaret Monteith and her husband, Matthew (profiled in *The Cut*, September 2016), discussed the series of financial events they went through to achieve a pregnancy. Not only did it take nine rounds of IVF and seven miscarriages, but they also sought new jobs in Massachusetts so they could profit from the state's coverage. In Massachusetts the coverage level is at 99 percent, the highest in the nation, and according to law, insurers must provide for AI; for IVF and ICSI; and for donor sperm, egg, or embryo procurement and processing. Medication coverage is handled just like medication for any other health problem plus there is no limit to the number of treatment cycles and no cap on expenditures.

INSURANCE FOR SPECIAL POPULATIONS

Low Income

ART remains a high purchase for a large proportion of nonwhite minority patients with low incomes. These women and those without health insurance are less likely to go to a doctor for fertility assistance. (Remember: only one-third of infertile women actively seek treatment.) When they do, a large proportion of nonwhite insurees must deal with racial prejudices, the high cost of treatment, difficulty understanding medical terminology and procedures, and additional cultural expectations and stigmas. Studies show that IVF use is closely associated with higher socioeconomic status since the economic cost of IVF plays a large role in the decision to pursue treatment or not.

Male Donors

All 50 states have passed laws ensuring that sperm donors remain anonymous and free of parental rights and duties. As for out-of-pocket expenses, a study of 111 male participants in *Urology Practice* (July 2016) showed that 47 percent reported financial strain to the point that they used their savings or went into debt. According to the *Asian Journal of Andrology* (2016), more states should offer mandates for male infertility.

Of the 15 states providing coverage for female infertility, only eight states mention male infertility. Two states—Montana and West Virginia—have laws that mandate coverage for undefined fertility services in Health Maintenance Organization (HMO) plans, and six states—California, Connecticut, Massachusetts, New Jersey, New York, and Ohio—also have laws that mandate some form of male coverage.

In California insurance companies must offer employers various plans that include infertility coverage for men, but employers are not required to offer those plans to their employees. Connecticut law states that insurance plans must cover diagnosis and treatment for individuals unable to conceive, and in Ohio, only HMO plans provide coverage to men. Massachusetts, New Jersey, and New York offer the most comprehensive coverage for male infertility care, with Massachusetts including coverage for sperm harvesting and banking for the diagnosis and treatment of testicular failure.

LGBT Population

Access is not any easier for LGBT populations. New Jersey's insurance laws did not help four lesbians who wanted to start a family, according to *Mother Jones* (Liss-Schultz, August 2016). The women were forced to sue the state after being denied insurance coverage for infertility treatments. They could not prove they engaged in two years of unprotected sexual intercourse for the purposes of conception. But now with Obamacare in a state of flux (as of this writing), no one knows what will happen. The prohibition of insurance policies based on sexual orientation may still prevail with discrimination against same-sex couples because they cannot get pregnant via their partners.

Another legal challenge affects homosexual couples like Sean Smith and Kale Taylor, who paid more than $20,000 for a fertility procedure using a surrogate mother. They assumed they would have to pay all expenses, but now they are pushing to make Hawaii the first state to require coverage for surrogates. (Hawaii is one of eight states that require insurance companies to cover IVF, but since the mandate applies only to married heterosexual couples, this discriminates against the LGBT community and single women.) In 2017, Smith and Taylor borrowed money and refinanced a second mortgage. Kaiser Permanente Hawaii objected to the proposed legislative bill, saying it would raise costs for the company and its customers. The Hawaii proposal passed the state senate in 2017, but unfortunately it died in the House.

INSURANCE FROM EMPLOYERS

Fertility services are becoming popular in the United States as employee perks, according to a survey in *Employee Benefit News* (Eisenberg, September 2016). Four percent of employers with fewer than 50 employees offer fertility services, and nearly 25 percent of larger companies offer fertility services to their employees as part of the overall healthcare package, but only 27 percent of U.S. private-sector employers provide ART coverage.

Fertility services are more common among employers with at least 500 employees. Twenty-six percent of those companies offer insurance coverage for IVF, and 60 percent of employers with more than 500 workers offer some type of fertility benefit although it can be limited to a consultation with a doctor. About one-third of those employers cover fertility drug therapy, 24 percent cover IVF, and 23 percent cover AI. Thirty-two percent of the mega-employers (those having 20,000-plus employees) cover ART in their insurance packages. In any case, research in 2018 by Willis Towers Watson—a global advisory, broking and solutions company—shows the percentage of employers offering fertility benefits is expected to grow from 55 percent in 2017 to 66 percent by 2019.

The International Council on Infertility Information Dissemination lists companies offering fertility-related employee benefits. These include Abbott, Ace Hardware, Kinkos, and Marriott. Nineteen percent cover IVF treatments, 12 percent cover fertility medication, and 9 percent cover non-IVF fertility treatments. Six percent cover visits with counselors, and 4 percent cover egg harvesting or freezing services, according to *Employee Benefit News* (Eisenberg, September 2016).

While most medical plans set a maximum coverage ceiling, some fertility solution vendors like Progyny, Inc. are attempting to change the way these benefits are offered. Karin Ajmani, president of healthcare services at Progyny, says her company's mission is to increase access to more comprehensive benefits so that women can achieve pregnancy faster using the best and most appropriate technology. Her belief is that if you devote more money toward a fertility benefit up front, companies can avoid some high-risk maternity expenses such as preterm birth (often related to a high multiple rate in IVF).

Recently more companies are starting to come on board and expand coverage. Intel, for example, in 2016 quadrupled its fertility benefit coverage to $40,000 and $20,000 in drugs, and other companies (not only technology producers but also telecommunications, media, retail, and school districts) like Cisco offer a $15,000 lifetime maximum for medical treatment and $10,000 for drugs.

Only 8 of the 15 states with fertility provisions mandate IVF coverage, according to RESOLVE, and to be fair, its cost can easily deter employers.

There are exceptions such as Southwest Airlines where employees are covered at 50 percent coinsurance for up to a $10,000 lifetime maximum of medical expenses for fertility treatment (after meeting a $500 deductible). Prescription drugs related to those treatments are covered at 50 percent coinsurance for up to a $5,000 lifetime maximum. More than 100 Southwest employees use this benefit annually.

The United States still has much to learn about health coverage from other countries. Take, for instance, Iran. The *International Journal of Fertility and Sterility* (Jafarzadeh-Kenarsari et al., April–June 2015) reported that participants in Iran exhibit a high demand for financial support from family and acquaintances as well as cooperation from insurance companies, governmental authorities, and nongovernmental entities. Also, in a 2001–2002 experimental study in Israel at Sheba Medical Center, when couples were offered free ART (Lande et al., *Fertility and Sterility*, February 2011), 90 percent of them achieved a live birth within four years. In short, when IVF is paid by the government or another public entity, very few couples discontinue treatment before a live birth is achieved.

VETERANS' INSURANCE

During a firefight in Afghanistan in 2005, Army Cpl. Tyler Wilson, then 20, had a bullet pierce his spine and leave him paralyzed below the waist. Since then, the Department of Veterans Affairs has given him free health care, as it does for all veterans disabled while in the military. Yet by law, the Department of Veterans Affairs could not then provide IVF, not even to a veteran whose ability to have children was impaired by an injury sustained in the line of duty.

In 2016 all that changed. The VA passed a law covering IVF for wounded veterans. As NPR tells it, Congress reversed the "infertility" law and filled the gap in insurance. In 2013 Tricare began covering 9.5 million active duty beneficiaries for 1,200 ART cycles at an out-of-pocket cost of less than $7,000 per cycle. It now fully covers ART for wounded warriors and severely injured service members suffering from posttraumatic stress disorder (PTSD) or damaged spinal cords.

For younger troops, the U.S. Defense Department came up with a twenty-first-century high-tech solution: freezing sperm and eggs. The Pentagon estimates that this storage program could cost about $150 million over five years and will be offered through Tricare. RESOLVE also provides grants, scholarships, and discounted programs for active duty military and veteran families.

NONPROFITS AND FERTILITY FUNDS

To address fertility needs, RESOLVE recommends creating a financial plan that prioritizes short-term and long-term goals. The latter should include retirement needs, appropriate and affordable insurance protection, adequate cash reserves, and the limitation of consumer credit card debt. In general, RESOLVE advises utilizing a home equity line of credit rather than a credit card to pay for ART. To use this option, RESOLVE gives strategic advice on refinancing a home at a lower rate.

Also, RESOLVE endorses hiring a financial planner. The best way to find a financial planner is through referrals from friends, colleagues, and others in similar situations. Couples also can consult organizations such as the Financial Planning Association and Certified Financial Planner Board of Standards as well as banks and other lending institutions.

CONCLUSION

High-tech fertility procedures can come with hefty price tags. Unless the intended parents live in Massachusetts or are military veterans, they usually have a sizeable amount of out-of-pocket expenses even if employers pick up some of the treatment costs or they live in a state that offers some ART coverage.

Mandated insurance has not yet kept up with the need for infertility treatment (only 15 states offer any coverage at all), but good budgeting, safe loans, and grants can help couples finance IVF and other ART procedures.

Consider following the cost-saving trend to eSET or single embryo transfer and PGD. Also, smart couples should evaluate the need for endometrial surgery and see if they qualify for innovative devices like INVO-Cell and IVF in a Box. Intended parents should also consult advocacy organizations like RESOLVE and SART for hints on lowering ART costs and taking advantage of refund programs.

Affording and succeeding in high-tech treatment is basic to moving closer to the goal of growing a family, but as Chapter 4 points out, legal issues can complicate fertility treatments. The lack of legislative regulations forces states to manage ART procedures through case law instead of through commonsense federal and state rulings.

CHAPTER 4

Legalities of ART

Ruby Torres, 36, always wanted a child, but in June 2014 tests revealed she had breast cancer. Before undergoing chemotherapy and radiation, she got married and signed a contract for in vitro fertilization (IVF) treatment. The IVF procedure resulted in seven embryos that she stored at a fertility bank. Meanwhile the marriage ended, and based on the contract that the couple signed, Ruby's ex-husband was not compelled to agree to having the embryos transferred to his ex-spouse, thus becoming a parent. Ruby contested that.

In August 2017 at Arizona Family Court, Judge Renee Korbin Steiner decided that the husband's rights (his financial obligations for a child and how a child might affect any inheritance) outweighed his former wife's rights to procreate and her desire to have a biologically related child. After listening to each side's arguments, the judge ordered that the embryos be donated to a third party such as a fertility bank or another couple. Now Ruby and her ex-spouse worry that a third party could go after them for monies should the embryos produce diseases or disabilities.

The above is the type of legal problems Assisted Reproductive Technology (ART) can create. In this chapter some of the important ART-related state court decisions are presented due to the absence of state and federal laws. Not surprisingly the decisions are shaped by ethical, societal, and cultural values, and their content refers to consent forms, proprietary rights, gamete donors, and right of privacy. The chapter also includes some of the precedent-making legal rulings, which began with the New Jersey Baby M surrogacy case in 1986, and shows the development and evolution of reproductive law in the United States starting with the 1973 Uniform Parentage Act. The chapter aims to show ART couples, especially those arranging surrogacy, that they need to consult attorneys about their rights to biological material if they divorce; disposition forms; legal documentation of parental rights; and wills, trusts, and estate documents.

FEDERAL GOVERNMENTAL REGULATIONS

As presented previously, an Arizona couple's fight for embryo possession illustrates the inconsistency of infertility rulings that governments
have been forced to arrive at. Although some state regulations govern donations of embryos, eggs, and sperm as well as surrogacy, federal regulation is scant. In most instances the prevailing law comes from the state
where the child is born. For instance, Arizona lacks any law whatsoever
to provide guidance on frozen embryos. In the absence of a policy decision from the legislature, the judgment was left to the state court. (Other
states have laws that specify that unless spouses consent, they are not
considered parents of IVF children after a divorce.)

Licensing

With respect to licensing regulations, fertility physicians contend they
are not only licensed by state medical boards but also supervised by three
federal agencies: the Centers for Disease Control and Prevention (CDC),
the Food and Drug Administration (FDA), and the Centers for Medicare
and Medicaid Services (CMS). The latter agency implements the Clinical
Laboratory Improvement Act, which ensures high laboratory standards;
the CDC regulates ART through Public Law 102-493, and the FDA
addresses fertility drugs. While association with these agencies sounds
as if fertility treatment is well supervised, just the opposite is true, and
patients need to research prospective clinics carefully before they undergo
procedures or write checks in payment.

No National Mandate

Promulgated in 1992 as the Fertility Clinic Success Rate and Certification Act (FCSRCA) in conjunction with Federal Trade Commission legislation, the Success and Certification Act is not a national mandate. It was
written into law to allay concerns about false advertising by fertility clinics and other patient advocacy issues. It is the only national legislation
regarding ART. According to the Success Rate Act, fertility clinics must,
at least since 1997, submit key data such as patients' infertility diagnoses,
information on the ART procedure used, and statistics on pregnancies and
births.

The Society for Assisted Reproductive Technology (SART) and CDC
collect this annual clinical data on treatment types and outcomes per cycle
on the CDC website, and the information covers more than 95 percent of
the nearly 500 U.S. clinics. In 2001 the CDC also established the States
Monitoring ART (SMART) Collaborative, which links state data on pregnancy outcomes to ART success rates. In 2002 the CDC published the first
ART surveillance summary, and in 2006 the CDC formed the National
ART Surveillance System (NASS) in conjunction with patient advocacy

organizations: RESOLVE, Path2Parenthood, Livestrong Fertility, the American Bar Association (ABA), American Society for Reproductive Medicine (ASRM), and SART. This information can be accessed online (see resources at end). By calculating standardized success rates for each clinic, NASS gives potential ART users an idea of their average chance of success. Each state's status is also listed on the ASRM website.

Outside of these annual compulsory federal summaries, the fertility industry is self-regulated by professional organizations. For instance, the ASRM Practice Committee issues guidelines on minimal standards for providing ART, informed consent, and the number of embryos for transference. The latest ASRM Guidelines on the Number of Embryos Transferred was released in 2009 when the committee recommended transferring no more than two embryos at a time to women under age 35.

At that time the ASRM also recommended requiring an insurance mandate for all states to ensure safety for both mothers and babies since the data show that states not offering insurance for infertility lead to a high number of embryos being transferred, resulting in many high-order, risky multiple births. This insurance goal for a national mandate has not been achieved yet.

The Debate on Regulation

Why is there so little regulation over a billion-dollar industry? The Pew Charitable Trusts (Ollove, March 18, 2015) explains why states are not eager to regulate ART. The reason comes down to money. The entrepreneurial or business lobby influences legislative activity on fertility treatments. Except for a 2015 law passed by the Utah legislature regarding ART and giving children conceived via sperm donation access to the medical histories of their biological fathers, a state law relating to ART is a rarity.

Due to the infertility industry's conflation of medicine and mercantilism, most aspects of ART still go unregulated, such as how many children may be conceived from one donor, what types of medical information must be supplied by donors, what genetic tests may be performed on embryos, how many fertilized eggs may be placed in a woman, and how old a donor can be.

Despite these omissions, the ASRM refuses to concede that professional groups take a hands-off approach to regulation. Instead fertility organizations point to licensing requirements and the fact that the federal government regulates all drugs and medical devices as well as the reproductive tissues used in ART. Compared, however, to countries such as Canada, the United Kingdom, Sweden, Germany, and Australia, the United States passes few regulations, says the Pew Charitable Trusts. In 2013 a Pew Research Center poll found that 12 percent of adults in the United States think IVF is wrong, 33 percent call it acceptable, and 46 percent are indifferent, according to the *Pacific Standard* (Judd, September 28, 2015).

Opinions on IVF, embryos, and genetic techniques are so diverse because they are too close to the taint of abortion and eugenics for many people's comfort, says Arthur Caplan, director of medical ethics at New York University's Langone School of Medicine. Caplan says antiregulatory sentiments are present in many states and even among members of the ASRM because ART evolved as a business, not a research enterprise.

More regulation in ART will probably have to come from consumers—those who have gone through the process or resulted from it. One such person is Lisa Swanson, a lawyer who learned at age 30 that she was donor conceived. When she tried to delve into information about her biological father, she was faced with an impasse—a situation that state regulation could have and should have corrected.

Surrogacy Laws—Federal Input

There are no federal laws regarding either gestational or traditional surrogacy. Instead, most surrogacy issues are determined by state courts and legislatures. (Gestational surrogacy evolved at first for women who could not carry a baby due to physical problems; now it is the procedure of choice for couples, singles, and same-sex couples.) That is why each state has an eclectic mix of legislation and case law pertaining to surrogacy. However, the U.S. Constitution trumps any state surrogacy laws since the Constitution expressly states that a person has the right to make decisions related to his or her body. Thus, the intended parents cannot force a surrogate to end the pregnancy for any reason, and the intended parents must accept custody of the child regardless of any disability.

As pointed out previously, Congress has passed exactly one federal statute dealing with ART: the Fertility Clinic Success Rate and Certification Act (1992). Regardless of what many people think, the FDA does not regulate ART. IVF-used drugs never passed through the FDA application process—they have off-label use as fertility enhancers but are not specifically for IVF.

More recently, however, third-party reproduction has come under the watchful eye of the FDA through the Current Good Tissue Practice Requirements (May 2005). These regulations govern human cells, tissues, and cellular and tissue-based products. Because sperm and eggs from two parties are utilized and implanted into the uterus of a person who is not a sexually intimate partner of either party who donates the sperm or the egg, the FDA requires eggs and sperm to be screened to the same level of safety that any tissue would be screened prior to transplantation such as a heart or lung. Physicians must guarantee that the donated biological tissues are 100 percent safe and protected against infectious diseases like hepatitis B, hepatitis C, and HIV.

Uniform Parentage Act of 1973

Several decades ago to encourage legal consistency among the states, the National Conference of Commissioners on Uniform State Laws approved the Uniform Parentage Act (UPA) in 1973. The act consented to artificial insemination (AI, at least in married couples), designating the husband as the father. As a recommendation, the act has no legal force and has never been universally adopted or adopted in the same way by the 19 states that incorporated it.

The rules, however, have been important in establishing broad social acceptance of donor AI and have made possible the opening of the first sperm banks to store and sell for AI. The rules establish parentage, thus bringing order to surrogate relationships, according to a Trinity College Senior Thesis by Makenzie B. Russo (Spring 2016). Before that, Darra L. Hofman in 2009 assembled a state-by-state survey of surrogacy laws (*William Mitchell Law Review*).

The UPA declares equal rights for children regardless of their parents' marital status. Juveniles require this because establishing parentage entitles children to secure certain benefits such as Social Security, veterans' benefits, and inheritance rights. The act also establishes legal parentage for children conceived by a method other than sexual intercourse (e.g., ART) and possibly carried by a woman other than the legal mother (surrogacy). The act continues to mandate the identification of natural fathers so that child support obligations may be ordered. It also focuses on legislation regarding parentage, paternity actions, and child support.

In 2000, the Uniform Law Commission revised the UPA and added a proposal by the National Conference of Commissioners on Uniform State Law on the acceptance of surrogacy agreements. The act was again amended in 2002 as a response to inconsistencies between states and their requirements for surrogacy contracts.

Article 8 of the act addresses gestational surrogacy agreements and incorporates parts of the USCACA (Uniform Status of Children of Assisted Conception Act). In 2008 the ABA created the Model Act Governing Assisted Reproductive Technology as a response to the inconsistencies resulting from legal issues relative to ART. The act was co-sponsored by several ABA sections: Individual Rights and Responsibilities; Real Property, Trust and Estate Law; Science and Technology Law; Young Lawyers Division; and the Health Law (Section of Family Law). Its purpose is to minimize exploitation of persons coping with infertility as well as those working with it by setting guidelines that many unregulated and unlicensed industries involved in ART can follow.

Cases of fraud, theft, and coercion have been prevented by this act. For example, in 2015, a California-based agency owner cheated a client out of approximately $270,000, and the owner was sentenced to 18 months in prison. Because of this and other cases, the Model Act requires agencies to obtain a license as an effort toward fair and ethical practice in ART. However, these laws are not binding and are intended only to guide states as they formulate their own laws.

STATE REGULATIONS

To date, although 17 states have statutes that regulate surrogacy, little uniformity is found. Furthermore in 21 states there is neither a law nor a published case regarding surrogacy, according to Diane Hinson, a Washington, D.C., lawyer who specializes in ART. According to *Stateline* (March 18, 2015) and George Washington University law professor Naomi Cahn, donor-conceived children should at least have access to full medical information about their biological parents. States generally determine surrogacy issues. For example, the Michigan courts reviewed a surrogate broker business and concluded that its commercial surrogacy was similar to commercial adoption and thus illegal. On the other hand, Kentucky courts ruled in a 1986 case that surrogacy did not constitute baby-selling if the contract was entered before conception.

New Jersey followed Michigan's lead in the former's infamous Baby M case in which the New Jersey Supreme Court invalidated the 1985 surrogacy agreement between the prospective parents. In this case the Sterns (wife Betsy Stern had multiple sclerosis) and surrogate Mary Beth Whitehead ended up in court when Whitehead decided that she did not want to give up all rights to her genetic child. The New Jersey court found that the Stern-Whitehead contract represented the sale of a child or, at the very least, the sale of a mother's right to her child. The court awarded Mr. Stern primary custody and concluded it was in the best interests of the child that Mary Beth Whitehead retained parental and visitation rights.

Not surprisingly, some state courts and legislatures continue to rule against commercial surrogacy agreements, using adoption law to rule that surrogacy compensation is an illegitimate payment for a child. Other state courts such as California permit gestational surrogacy and have begun to establish a set of rights for parents who contract with a gestational carrier. In Maine gestational surrogacy is permitted and regulated under the Maine Parentage Act (Title 19-A 1932). It was previously sanctioned by case law in *Nolan v. Labree* in 2012. The genetic parents were permitted to be listed on the birth certificate of a child born to a gestational surrogate. The reasoning followed a 2011 statute that provided for the district court to declare "parentage" a term that included both paternity and maternity. Therefore, the district court had the authority to declare the maternity of the female genetic parent (Columbia Law School, Sexuality and Gender Law Clinic, May 2016).

State statutes pertaining to surrogacy are especially diverse since a third actor—the pregnancy carrier—now comprises the treatment plan, bringing with her a unique set of emotional, social, and economic motives. For instance, some hormonal changes during pregnancy produce a maternal instinct in the pregnant surrogate, and that situation can exacerbate the separation process upon birth (Jon Sterngass, *Reproductive Technology*, Benchmark Books, 2011). Another difficulty is the discovery through amniocentesis of a genetic abnormality in the fetus such as Down syndrome, at which time the surrogate may refuse to abort the fetus. These events and the powerful responses they evoke in people contribute toward the reason that much of Europe bans the practice of surrogacy, and 12 states, including New Jersey, New York, and Michigan, refuse to recognize surrogacy contracts. Other states, including Texas, California, Pennsylvania, and Florida, have legalized and regulated the process.

On the other hand, seven states have at least one court opinion upholding some form of surrogacy, with California having the most permissive laws in the country. In general, restrictions (or the lack thereof) of surrogacy laws are due to concerns about the divisive subject of abortion. In Louisiana, for example, this politically conservative state allows only altruistic surrogacy.

Surrogate Brokers

Because surrogacy is not well regulated, couples are encouraged to do due diligence when screening potential surrogates and surrogate agencies. This prevents later legal and emotional misunderstandings and complications. To minimize this, prospective surrogates should demonstrate the following attributes:

- Responsibility
- Employment of surrogate or partner
- A supportive partner
- Well-established community roots
- A helpful attitude and belief that money is secondary
- No drug history
- A track record of keeping appointments with doctors, lawyers, and prospective intended parents
- Has a regular obstetrician-gynecologist
- Asks good questions and signs paperwork only after reading it.

(Adapted from the *ABA Guide to Assisted Reproduction: Techniques, Legal Issues, and Pathways to Success*)

ART LAWYERS

The messy state of ART regulation should motivate intended parents to find an ART-certified lawyer. Couples should be able to locate an ART attorney in their area since the American Bar Association (ABA) has expanded to include a surrogacy and reproductive technology section. As a result, ART attorneys in different states are knowledgeable about the laws in their specific geographic locales.

Couples can contact an attorney through the American Academy of Assistive Reproductive Technology Attorneys in Washington, D.C. The following questions from the *ABA Guide to Assisted Reproduction* can aid in selection:

1. Where is the ART attorney licensed? If the surrogate expects to give birth outside the attorney's jurisdiction, then this lawyer cannot help you!
2. What is the cost or retainer? What about additional costs such as court filing fees, copies, or other administrative fees?
3. Does the lawyer charge a flat fee or bill hourly?
4. Does the lawyer's firm offer other needed legal services such as tax law, trusts, and estate services or immigration?
5. What percentage of the lawyer's practice is ART law?
6. Will the intended parents be working directly with a lawyer or a legal staff member? What is the lawyer's accessibility?

A specialized lawyer is not a luxury when it comes to surrogate arrangements. As with countries, individual states view surrogacy contracts between prospective parents and egg donors with idiosyncratic attitudes.

SURROGACY CONTRACTS IN THE UNITED STATES

In the absence of specific statutory guidance by the UPA, when parties to an ART agreement disagree, courts must determine the legal parentage of the children on a case-by-case basis, and it is entirely unclear how binding such contracts would be.

For instance, in five states, surrogacy contracts are void and unenforceable. Arizona and Indiana also invalidate all surrogacy agreements by statute. In addition to declaring surrogacy agreements void, some jurisdictions impose civil or criminal penalties. The District of Columbia imposes a civil penalty up to $10,000 and a criminal penalty of up to one-year imprisonment on anyone who facilitates a surrogacy contract.

The most notorious example of a failed surrogacy contract is in the New Jersey Baby M case (previously mentioned). In more recent cases, New Jersey courts have not followed the Baby M precedent that discriminated between traditional and gestational surrogacy agreements. For example, in *A.G.R. v. D.R.H.* (2009), a gay male couple in New Jersey entered into a gestational surrogacy contract with D.R.'s sister. After giving birth to twins who bore no genetic relation to the sister, she filed suit to retain parental rights and to void the contract she had with D.R. and S.H. The couple moved for a summary judgment, claiming that because the sister had no genetic link to the children, the case was different from Baby M. Ultimately the court held that the sister would retain her parental rights, and the contract was void.

The lack of surrogacy laws has left participants at a strong disadvantage because the inconsistency in state regulations artificially limits the supply of surrogacy agencies, medical specialists, and gestational surrogates, further increasing costs. Attempts have been made to improve the system, but none go far enough to ensure that each party will be fully protected and aware of the potential outcomes. One thing everyone does agree on is the need for a legislative instrument to eliminate the confusion, ambiguity, and unpredictability that currently exist.

International Surrogacy

On an international level, Kim Cotton's 1985 case became Britain's first commercial surrogate mother case to emphasize the ethical and legal issues at stake in a debate about motherhood and parenthood. Cotton bore a child for an American couple, but upon birth, the court claimed the baby as a ward for the state until a determination was made as to its parentage.

As already pointed out, some countries have ART regulations, but an opinion in the Brooklyn *Journal of Policy and Law* (2016) proposed that a Hague International Convention should regulate international surrogacy agreements using a method like the proposed 2010 Indian Assisted Reproductive Technology (Regulation) Bill and Rules or Israel's 2012 Expert Committee Recommendations. The opinion recommended that regulation in various countries could be modeled after Israeli legislation or proposed Indian regulations because both these documents helped address the risks and pitfalls of international surrogacy and protected the future thousands of parents and surrogates as well as the resulting children.

Legal Precedents in the United States

Divorce

In *Davis v. Davis* (1992), the Supreme Court of Tennessee decided a dispute over cryopreserved pre-embryos in favor of Junior Lewis Davis, who wanted to destroy the pre-embryos over the objections of his ex-wife. The *Davis* decision, though not binding in other states, suggested a model framework for similar disputes: U.S. courts should follow the wishes of those who contribute their sperm and egg cells to create pre-embryos.

A.Z. v. B.Z. was a 2000 case heard by the Massachusetts Supreme Court that focused on a prior written agreement to the disposition of frozen embryos in the event of a divorce. The court decided that the agreement was unenforceable. This is the first reported case in which a court decided not to enforce an agreement that compelled one donor to become a parent against his or her will.

In *J.B. v. M.B.* (2001), the Supreme Court of New Jersey decided a dispute between a divorced couple over cryopreserved IVF pre-embryos. The former wife (J.B.) wanted the pre-embryos destroyed while her ex-husband (M.B.) wanted them for future implantation such as by an infertile couple. The court declined to force J.B. to become a parent against her will, concluding that doing so would violate state public policy.

In re Marriage of Witten (2003), the Iowa Supreme Court held that neither Tamera nor Arthur Witten could use or destroy several cryopreserved pre-embryos created for IVF during their marriage unless the couple could reach an agreement.

Wrongful Life

Paretta v. Medical Offices for Human Reproduction was a 2003 case heard by the Supreme Court of New York. It dealt with a child born with cystic fibrosis due to the IVF doctors failing to disclose that the egg donor was a known carrier of cystic fibrosis genes. The doctors also failed to test Mr. Paretta's sperm to determine if he was a carrier. The court decided that a child cannot sue on a theory of wrongful life, but the parents can sue for medical expenses incurred now and in the future due to the doctors' negligence.

Proprietary Rights

In the case *York v. Jones* (1989), the U.S. District Court for the Eastern District of Virginia was one of the first U.S. courts to address a dispute over a cryopreserved pre-embryo. Married couple Steven York and Risa Adler-York provided gametes to doctors who then created the pre-embryo at the Howard and Georgeanna Jones Institute for Reproductive Medicine in Norfolk, Virginia. The institute refused to relinquish possession of the pre-embryos, claiming their proprietary rights were limited to implantation, donation to another infertile couple, donation for approved research, or thawing. An interinstitutional transfer was not an option. The court found that the couple had property rights, as claimed under the agreement, and could repossess the pre-zygotes and were thus entitled to compensation.

In Missouri, *McQueen v. Gadberry* (2016) was a case of disputed authority over cryopreserved embryos in a divorce. The litigation was unique in that it attempted to classify the embryos as persons. The appeals court affirmed the trial court's judgment that the embryos were marital property that the husband and wife both held rights to and would have to agree on as to their disposition. The argument that the pre-embryos were children was found to have no merit.

Consent Forms

In *Maureen Kass v. Steven Kass* (1998) the Court of Appeals of New York in Albany ruled that the state should generally consider IVF consent forms signed by participants in an IVF program (including handling cryo-preserved pre-zygotes or pre-embryos) to be valid, binding, and enforceable in the event of a dispute.

In *Randy M. Roman v. Augusta N. Roman* (2006) the Court of Appeals of Texas modeled their decision after the courts in other states and upheld the validity and enforceability of IVF consent agreements. Married in July 1997, the Romans visited the Center for Reproductive Medicine in Clear Lake, Texas, in August 2001. Doctors tried AI three times but failed, and the Romans agreed to IVF. In March 2002 the Romans signed a document in which they agreed to allow the center to cryopreserve the pre-embryos until they were ready to be transferred to Augusta. The Romans also agreed to allow the center to discard any cryopreserved pre-embryos should they later divorce.

Doctors extracted 13 eggs from Augusta and fertilized 6. Although Augusta was scheduled to have the three resulting pre-embryos transferred later that month, Randy withdrew his consent the night before the procedure. The pre-embryos remained in cryopreservation.

The now-divorced Romans each sought different outcomes. Randy wanted the embryos destroyed; Augusta wanted them implanted. The Texas court, citing several related cases, declared that the written IVF consent form the Romans had signed would govern the outcome. In February 2004 the trial court concluded that the pre-embryos were community property and awarded them to Augusta, a decision the court regarded as fair and equitable.

Randy then appealed this decision, arguing that the trial court should have enforced the agreement the Romans had signed to discard the frozen pre-embryos in the event of divorce. Given that there was no Texas case law addressing the enforceability of IVF consent forms, the appellate court surveyed cases from other states about frozen pre-embryo disputes (see cases discussed previously). Finally, the Texas court looked at *Litowitz v. Litowitz* (2002), a Washington State case that enforced a provision to destroy the pre-embryos after five years in cryopreservation. The Texas court also looked at an Iowa decision in *In re Marriage of Witten* (2003) that neither party could use their pre-embryos without mutual consent.

In 2001 the Texas court passed the UPA. Using this as a model, the court determined that Texas policy allowed a couple to determine in advance what should happen to their pre-embryos in the case of divorce.

In February 2006 the Texas Court of Appeals ruled that the Romans' consent agreement to discard the pre-embryos should have been honored.

In the 2008 court case *In the Matter of the Marriage of Dahl and Angle*, the Court of Appeals of Oregon upheld a written IVF consent form signed by a married couple who each contributed their genetic material to several pre-embryos. The court decision followed the general finding by the Supreme Court of Tennessee in *Davis v. Davis* in 1992 (see above), a decision subsequently followed by many courts across the United States.

Right of Privacy

In the case of *David J. Litowitz v. Becky M. Litowitz* (2002) Washington State reached a decision that neither party wanted. David sought to find adoptive parents for two cryopreserved pre-embryos created during his marriage to Becky. Becky sought to implant the pre-embryos in a surrogate so she might parent a child. The court found that the privacy interest (right of privacy in procreative choice) in David's reproductive function under both the U.S. and Washington State constitutions compelled the award of the pre-embryo to David Litowitz.

Wrongful Death/Personhood

In *Jeter v. Mayo* (2005) the Court of Appeals of Arizona held that a cryopreserved three-day-old pre-embryo is not a person and that the Arizona legislature was best suited to decide whether to expand the law to include cryopreserved pre-embryos. It affirmed a decision by the Maricopa County Superior Court to dismiss the couple's wrongful death claim after the Mayo Clinic allegedly lost or destroyed several of their cryopreserved pre-embryos.

This case was the first of its kind to address questions of personhood in an IVF-created human embryo. It established the importance of prior written agreements for disposition of frozen embryos. The court decided that Thomas Doolan's identity or personhood existed at the embryo stage. The fact that he was born with cystic fibrosis was not attributable to the decision of the IVF providers to implant one embryo instead of another. The other unused embryo may not have carried the cystic fibrosis genes, but that other embryo was not Thomas Doolan. The decision in Doolan has not been publicly tested in other jurisdictions.

Contract

Daryl Hendrix v. Samantha Harrington (2006) is a case of a gay Kansas man who decided that despite a written document, he wanted joint custody of the twins he fathered. The dispute centered on a 1994 statute that says a donor of semen used in AI of a woman other than his wife is treated as though he is not the birth father of a child unless the donor and woman agree to it in writing. The father was denied custody by the Kansas Supreme Court, which ruled that without a written contract, sperm donors were not legal parents and did not possess parental rights. Hendrix appealed to the U.S. Supreme Court, but the judges declined to hear the case.

Posthumous

In 2011 an Israeli court set a global precedent by allowing the family to harvest their dead daughter's eggs. The critical issue, according to the Mount Sinai School of Medicine in New York, was whether the daughter would have wanted her biological child to come to life after she was dead. Ethicist Arthur Caplan said that the laws and policies need to catch up with practices. The Israeli court approved the extraction and fertilization of the eggs.

Gamete Donors

Sperm donors in the United States generally provide the biological content for reproduction but give up all legal rights over the children. Also, American law usually protects sperm donors from responsibilities relating to the children. But some court cases minimize these protections. In 1991 *Anna Johnson v. Mark Calvert* was heard by the California Court of Appeals since the surrogate decided she had rights as a parent and filed for custody. Because the surrogate was black and not wealthy, and the contracting couple was white and well off, controversy was stirred. However, after a decision that favored the couple, the California Court of Appeals held that the appellant was not the natural mother of the child since the results of blood tests excluded her as the genetic mother. It ruled that under California law, the person who supplied the egg was the natural mother and the person who supplied the sperm was the natural father. In California, therefore, the courts tied "intent" to motherhood when genetic links and labor did not coincide in the same woman.

In *In the Interest of P.S., a Child* (2016) the Second District Court of Appeals of Texas ruled over a case in which a man provided his sperm to a female friend. He agreed it would be used for insemination, and a child was conceived. The man was involved with the child for a while until the mother refused him access and asked him to relinquish his right. He sought to be declared the father of the child, but Texas law required that if a man is to be considered a donor with no rights or responsibilities to the child, then his sperm must be provided to a licensed physician for use in ART. Since the man had never used a physician, the court held that he was a parent but not a donor.

Gay Rights

In 2008 the California Supreme Court heard the case of *North Coast Women's Care Medical Group v. Superior Court*. The key issue was whether physicians could use a religious freedom defense to refuse to perform an infertility treatment on a lesbian couple. The case involved Guadalupe Benitez, a resident of San Diego County. Due to the physician's refusal to render service to Benitez, she had to go outside her employer's medical network and pay for treatment without insurance coverage. The court ruled in favor of the plaintiff because the judges maintained that the physicians could have refused to perform the IUI procedure on all the clinic's patients or, more sensibly, could have used a doctor without religious objections. This case was perceived as a victory for gay rights in California.

In *Partanen v. Gallagher* the Massachusetts Supreme Judicial Court declared that Karen Partanen, a nonbirth mother, could be a legal parent to the two children she raised with her former partner Julie Gallagher. The two children were born using ART (GLAD Legal Advocates & Defenders for the LGBTQ Community, October 2016). In overturning the ruling that an unmarried gay woman does not have the same parental rights as the biological mother, the supreme judicial court found that a gay person may establish themselves as a child's presumptive parent under state law despite lacking a biological relationship.

The *State of Kansas et al. v. W.M. and A.B.*, tried in November 22, 2016, in Shawnee County, Kansas, involved a man who answered a Craigslist ad for a sperm donor. He provided his sperm to an unmarried lesbian couple and, without medical intervention, inseminated one of the partners. After the child was born, the partners separated, and the custodial mother applied for state benefits. The state sued for paternity determination and reimbursement of child support, but Kansas law requires medical involvement as a necessity to be considered a sperm donor. The court considered the best interests of the child and who had the stronger parental rights and responsibilities. The court held that the donor was not a parent and therefore had no duty to repay the state.

No Relationship

In *Lamaritata v. Lucas* on August 16,2002, the Florida Second District Court of Appeals found that the two unmarried parents did not constitute a couple since they had no relationship. Thus, the father should have no visitation rights. The court rejected a previous written agreement that granted Mr. Lucas visitation rights and maintained that he was only a sperm donor, not a parent entitled to visitation rights (*Florida Bar Journal*, 2014).

Conclusion

Compared to countries like Canada, Sweden, Germany, Australia, and the United Kingdom (Britain has a regulatory agency known as the Human Fertilisation and Embryo Authority, and Canada passed the 2004

Assisted Human Reproduction Act, which regulated the use of ART technologies), the United States is only lightly regulated in ART. Each state decides issues based on past cases and whatever legislation it may have adopted.

While the federal government regulates ART laboratories, neither the United States nor state governments do much to oversee the multibillion-dollar fertility industry. States are split over issues such as the advisability of surrogacy contracts, how many children can be conceived from one donor, what types of medical information or updates must be supplied by donors, what genetic tests may be performed on embryos, how many fertilized eggs may be placed in a woman, and how old a donor can be. States also have different attitudes regarding LBGT relationships and parentage. The maze of state laws, contracts, and court cases can easily befuddle the average person, but a competent ART-informed attorney can help steer intended parents in the right direction.

In the next chapter, laws and regulations take a back seat to physical and emotional challenges. Readers find out about the downside of ART—the injuries or diseases that can result from IVF and other fertility and gene-analysis techniques.

CHAPTER 5

Risks of ART

Every action in life is fraught with risks. Assisted Reproductive Technology (ART) is no exception. Although egg and sperm donors, physicians, intended parents, and surrogates hope for the best—a healthy baby and mother—oftentimes physical and emotional obstacles block the fertility procedure from producing the desired results. The risks for parents and children may be medical and/or mental, temporary or permanent, trivial or tremendous, but whatever their consequence, they must be acknowledged and dealt with. Part of that process is informed consent, which when done properly accords patients full knowledge of the risks and benefits. Sometimes, however, patients do not take informed consent seriously and neglect to factor in the downside of ART.

This chapter discusses that downside—the dangers that can befall prospective parents, such as postpartum depression, infections, and ovarian hyperstimulation syndrome (OHSS), and the unfortunate disorders ART children may encounter such as autism and cerebral palsy. Although fertility clinics and physicians do not want their patients to obsess over the risks, they are duty bound to discuss them and provide appropriate information through written documents and face-to-face questions and answers.

Let's first look at the challenges and dangers men face.

MALE RISKS AND POTENTIAL COMPLICATIONS
Weight

Paternal overweight or obesity can harm IVF treatment outcomes. During a study of 651 couples, including 345 men with a normal BMI (body mass index) and 306 men with an overweight BMI, the results showed that individuals with higher BMIs exhibited significantly lower fertilization rates compared to their normal BMI counterparts. The mean sperm telomere length (STL), which represents repetitive areas of DNA on chromosomes, was significantly shorter than that of the normal BMI groups. Research shows that STL is shorter in males who are infertile. The loss of telomere length results in the aging and death of male germ cells as well as the stopping of meiosis or cell division in female germ cells. These outcomes may partially account for obese men's poor treatment results in IVF cycles.

Emotions

Even though men do not experience the hormonal blasts from IVF medications that women do, they can become emotionally wrought. In *Marriage and Family Therapy* (Martins et al., March 2016) 12 studies from three continents yielded 2,534 records. The results revealed that psychological symptoms of maladjustment significantly increased in men one year after the first fertility evaluation.

According to Fertility Centers of Illinois, the stress of men not being able to procreate has been associated with emotional problems such as anger, depression, and feelings of worthlessness and anxiety over their potency, masculinity, and sexual adequacy. Additionally, marital problems and guilt can trigger or worsen erectile dysfunction, which in turn exacerbates the feelings of inadequacy that accompany infertility.

Male infertility is also frequently associated with high levels of stigma due to its perceived association with sexual dysfunction. Male factor infertility has attracted such social stigma and culture of secrecy that women sometimes take the blame for the couple's struggles, thus perpetuating their cycle of guilt and insecurity.

Surgical Sperm Retrieval

When men cannot provide enough sperm through masturbation, the recommended procedure is Surgical Sperm Retrieval (SSR). About 5–10 percent of IVF procedures involve SSR from the testes. Common side effects from the sedatives and narcotics are nausea and a lack of recall of the procedure. There also may be respiratory depression, which can reduce a person's oxygen level. More common are bleeding and infection. Men can feel uncomfortable for several days and need good scrotal support and an analgesic. Up to 80 percent of men undergoing SSR have inflammation or pooling of blood at the site of the biopsy.

Inflammation in the testes is likely to reduce future sperm production and damage blood vessels in the testes. Complete loss of blood supply and the atrophy of the testes has been reported after a testicular biopsy, but a repeated SSR procedure is more likely to be successful if done at least six months after the last procedure. This suggests that SSR probably causes temporary damage to the testes.

FEMALE RISKS AND POTENTIAL COMPLICATIONS

Women's risks derive from a combination of drugs and invasive procedures that can cause uncomfortable emotions and bloating as well as a fear of getting cancer.

Drugs

One drug in particular—Lupron—has had mixed results in inducing greater production of eggs. Originally developed for advanced prostate cancer, it is now commonly used to treat women with endometriosis and fibroids and to aid in ART procedures. Since 1999 the Food and Drug Administration (FDA) reports adverse drug reports on Lupron ranging from itching and dizziness to hypertension, muscular pain, and liver function abnormality. The FDA has not approved Lupron specifically for use in infertility or ART; its use is considered "off label" and at the discretion of the physician. The National Women's Health Network is concerned that no data have been gathered on Lupron's long-term effects for endometriosis, fibroids, or ART and wants to establish a registry to monitor the drug's effects on women and children. Cancer, of course, is the biggest fear (see below "cancer risk").

Venous Thromboembolism and Hysterectomy

ART increases the risk of venous thromboembolism (VTE) during super ovulation and pregnancy and the danger of an emergency peripartum hysterectomy to stop hemorrhaging after the birth of the baby.

Egg Harvesting

Procedures to gather women's eggs can lead to problems: infections, punctures of internal organs, hemorrhages, ovarian trauma, and intrapelvic adhesions. Up to 1 percent of women who undergo egg retrieval end up hospitalized, usually from complications of OHSS. Although the egg harvesting step of IVF is not major surgery, it is still surgery and entails risks. Even the anesthetic given for the procedure may cause a reaction.

Stress

Human Reproduction (Gameiro et al., August 2016) concludes that while most women show resilience after IVF treatments, 37 percent show temporary or chronic maladjustment.

Furthermore, in a 2016 doctoral dissertation at Walden University, the author says the stress of ART is equivalent to that in women with cancer, AIDS, or heart disease. Like PTSD (posttraumatic stress disorder), ART can disturb the patient's emotional equilibrium.

Psychological stress affects both women and men since the stress incorporates physical, financial, and emotional components. Experts try to minimize these effects through screening and online intervention, but in a study on personalized e-therapy programs between 2011 and 2013, women were monitored until three months after the start of their first ART cycle, and the findings were mixed. Most women declined participation in the study because they felt no need for support, but the online intervention was deemed effective judging by the reduction in the percentage of women having symptoms of anxiety and/or depression compared with those of the control group. The conclusion was that personalizing an e-therapy program to the fertility patients' risk profiles is a promising and feasible therapy (van Dongen et al., *Human Reproduction*, 2016).

Psychological adjustment after IVF failure (Gameiro, *Human Reproduction*, August 2016) has been studied long-term. Funded by the Hong Kong University Grant Council, the study found that regret was present only among participants with no remaining frozen embryos left for another cycle. Another study of 348 women (Gameiro, *Human Reproduction*, 2016) and their psychological resilience to IVF found that 86 percent of women showed normal levels of anxiety and depression throughout treatment. Higher levels were associated with unsuccessful treatment, marital dissatisfaction, lack of social support, and negative thoughts about infertility. One in 10 women had chronic anxiety 11–17 years after treatment. The *Journal of Psychology and Clinical Psychiatry* (Cassidy et al., 2016) published a study of 363 women undergoing ART and found that negative mental health effects can be neutralized by self-compassion, secure attachment, social support, and problem-focused and emotion-focused coping strategies.

Women with Antiphospholipid Syndrome, Lupus, and Ulcerative Colitis

In June 2015 the European League against Rheumatism announced that ART can be safely used in lupus and antiphospholipid syndrome (APS) if the disease is stable and in remission and preventive measures are used to limit the risk of flares or thrombosis (formation of a blood clot). According to a study of 37 women with lupus or APS who underwent 97 IVF procedures, the pregnancy rate was 28 percent and the live birth rate was 85 percent. These percentages were close to what is expected in the general population, which is why researchers maintain that IVF can be safely performed in women in remission with lupus and APS.

However, this prognosis is controversial because antiphospholipid antibodies are being detected more frequently in women undergoing IVF. Although their presence does not appear to influence the outcome, the available evidence concludes that antiphospholipid antibodies play some role in recurrent miscarriage, which is why these affected women are usually treated with aspirin and heparin (Heng et al., *Integrative Medicine International*, 2015).

A 20-year Danish study of women with ulcerative colitis (UC) showed that ART is less likely to work for these women. Investigators concluded that women with UC ought to initiate ART sooner than other women because they cannot expect the same success per embryo transfer. Also, there is a greater risk of preterm birth, at least for twins.

CANCER RISKS FOR WOMEN

Overall Risk

One of the biggest ART risks for women is cancer triggered by the various fertility drugs, but some doctors tend to gloss over this or paint a confusing or contradictory picture, leaving women unsure of their risk level. The American Society for Reproductive Medicine (ASRM) says the data so far seem to indicate no long-term problems, but Timothy Johnson, MD, chair of the University of Michigan's obstetrics and gynecology department, says there is a lack of information about the long-term effects. A 2013 meta-analysis of 25 studies found no convincing evidence of an increase in the risk of invasive ovarian cancer linked to the use of fertility drugs, but Northwestern University's fertility clinic suggests another possibility. Researchers there claim that although current evidence does not support a relationship between fertility drugs and an increased risk of cancer, no long-term research has been done to determine the risks of fertility drugs on breast, ovarian, and uterine cancer rates.

Perhaps long-term research would have helped college student Maggie Eastman. She donated her eggs 10 times between 2003 and 2013. The money attracted her, and risk awareness was not a priority given her youth. Maggie Eastman now considers ovarian donation to be the worst decision she ever made. In 2013 after her final egg donation, she was diagnosed with stage 4 metastatic breast cancer. Her oncologist could not discount the possibility that certain IVF drugs that increased her hormone production might have contributed to or caused her cancer.

Informed consent could be lacking for women. A 2010 study of 80 donors in *Fertility and Sterility* (between 1989 and 2002) in 20 states found that 20 percent of women said they did not know of any possible health risks at the time of their first egg donation. The coauthor of this study said that most women consider the procedure minor, and about 21 percent evaluate the risks as extremely minor. A total of 37 percent viewed the potential risks as serious and 11 percent indicated the risks as very serious.

Furthermore a 2014 study of egg donation advertisements placed on Craigslist found that most ads did not include risk information. Diane Tober, a medical anthropologist who interviewed 60 egg donors for a related film, said that some donors seemed naïve, expecting the fertility doctors to inform them thoroughly and monitor them closely during the process. Do some women miss out on informed consent altogether?

A 2016 study of 25,000 Dutch women may reconcile some of the older contradictory information on cancer. This large study not only found no increased risk among women receiving IVF but also found no greater risk among women who had various types of less intensive fertility treatments such as artificial insemination (AI). The researchers factored in many variables linked to higher risks of cancer, including the woman's age at the time she gave birth to her first child (IVF patients tend to have children later in life), her overall number of births, and the number of IVF attempts.

Still, the Dutch study is not conclusive, says the American Cancer Society. A national registry that tracks the health of IVF participants is warranted, say experts like Judy E. Stern, a Dartmouth professor who oversees the Infertility Family Research Registry, a voluntary database of 70 egg donors. Stern says Society for Assisted Reproductive Technology (SART) is considering establishing such an egg-donor registry to track IVF patients since most large fertility centers do not inform their women donors of the significant cancer risk. Ironically many of these same fertility centers who neglect to produce informational patient brochures are members of ASRM.

A 2013 editorial in *JAMA* called for more complete data on both short and long-term outcomes of egg donation, and a 2007 *New England Journal of Medicine* article warned that women must be ensured that their health is not compromised. The need for more data is partly based on anecdotal reports. For instance, Jennifer Schneider, MD, a Tucson-based internist, saw her daughter succumb to colon cancer diagnosed in 2003. Schneider attributes her daughter's death to her tenure as an egg donor.

Ovarian Cancer

Risk of reproductive cancers may exist for ART women due to ovarian stimulation drugs and increased hormone levels. Fortunately, the risk numbers are often very small, such as an increase from 1 percent to 2 percent. The following data support the case for long-term studies:

a. A 2011 Dutch study of 19,000 women concluded that ovarian stimulation may increase the risk of ovarian cancer, particularly borderline ovarian tumors.

b. A 2013 U.S. study of 9,825 women found that women who used ovulation-inducing drugs and did not become pregnant demonstrated a higher risk of ovarian cancer than those who became pregnant.

c. A 2013 retrospective study of 87,000 Israeli women found no significant relationship between IVF and the risks of breast, endometrial, or ovarian cancers but demonstrated a trend of an increased risk of ovarian cancer related to the number of IVF cycles the women underwent.

    d. A 2013 study of more than 21,000 Australian women found no evidence of increased risk of ovarian cancer following IVF in women who gave birth. In those who never gave birth, there was a marked increase in the risk of ovarian cancer.

    e. A 2015 study of more than 100,000 Israeli women found IVF treatments pose a significant risk of ovarian and uterine cancer.

    f. A 2015 ASRM conference at which researchers presented data from IVF studies of 250,000 British women between 1991 and 2010 compared their results to the general population. ART patients had a 30 percent greater likelihood of developing ovarian cancer.

Breast Cancer

Results here are also varied, which underscores the need for long-term studies.

    a. A 2012 Australian study of 21,000 women compared IVF patients with those receiving other fertility treatments. The result was an increased rate of breast cancer in women who commenced IVF at age 24 or younger.

    b. A 2014 U.S. study of more than 12,000 women found that women who used fertility drugs did not have an increased risk of breast cancer.

    c. A 2015 study of more than 800,000 Norwegian women who gave birth found that the risk of breast cancer was 20 percent higher for IVF-treated women than for those who got pregnant spontaneously.

    d. A 2016 Swedish study of more than 40,000 women aged 40–69 found that women who had undergone ovarian stimulation showed increased density of breast tissue, which is a risk factor for breast cancer.

Endometrial Cancer

A 2013 study of 12,000 women found a slightly elevated risk of endometrial cancer associated with two medications for ovarian stimulation—clomiphene and gonadotropins. Also, when Alastair Sutcliffe, MD, from the Institute of Child Health, University College London, and his team evaluated 255,786 records, they looked at many women who used ART from 1992 to 2010. The results were presented at the 2015 ASRM annual meeting and suggested that there was little for women to worry about regarding the risk of cancers from the IVF drug treatments they undergo.

The above cancer studies are inconsistent at best. Bias is always a possibility, especially in professional organizations like ASRM. Thus, it makes more sense for federal agencies like the NIH (National Institutes of Health) or Centers for Disease Control and Prevention (CDC) to conduct long-term studies to finally resolve the connection between cancer and IVF.

OTHER MEDICAL RISKS FOR WOMEN

OHSS

Most women have pain and discomfort during IVF, mainly from the hormones, but about 30 percent also experience bloating, cramping, mood swings, nausea, diarrhea, and abdominal pain or tenderness. Moderate OHSS provoked by hormones such as Clomiphene, Lupron, and Repronex can induce vomiting, rapid weight gain, increased size of the abdomen (from fluid retention), and decreased or no urination. OHSS requires bed rest and close monitoring of electrolytes, blood counts, and fluids. Women with a severe form of OHSS may suffer renal impairment, liver dysfunction, thromboembolic phenomena (a clot blocks a blood vessel), shock, and, in a few cases, adult respiratory distress syndrome. Severe cases can be complicated by the rupture of the ovaries or their twisting.

OHSS was the most common complication among 1,135,206 IVF cycles between 2000 and 2011 (Kawwass et al., *JAMA*, January 2015). No donor deaths were reported, but 13 maternal deaths prior to infant births were reported among egg donor recipients.

Multiple Pregnancies

Multiple births are dangerous for mothers. Women expecting multiples are also at risk for hypertension, postpartum hemorrhage, prolonged bed rest, and diabetes. Multiple pregnancies are common when implanting more than one or two embryos, especially with the increased risk of hormone therapy and older mothers' ages. Fully 5 percent of babies born to mothers in their late 30s are multiples, a figure that rises to 6 percent for babies born to mothers in their early 40s. For women 45 and older, one in five babies is a multiple (Livingston, Pew Research Center, National Center for Health Statistics, 2015b). Complications of ART from multiple pregnancies are common and can be prevented or minimized by limiting the number of embryos transplanted.

Besides, a 2011 study of births resulting from ART, researchers found that significant differences were obtained between groups of single birth and multiple birth families with respect to material necessities, social stigma, marital satisfaction, depression, and quality of life. Scientists concluded that having more than one child per birth increases the psychosocial risks for the parents and that psychological counseling should be included before initiating ART and when a multiple pregnancy is confirmed.

Mental Problems

In January 2011 *Human Reproduction Update* (Ross et al.) published results of a review of 13 articles on postpartum psychosis (PPP) following

ART. The results concluded that PPP often co-occurs in multiple births. Consequently, it is hard to separate those two variables. In another small study of 63 ART patients and 72 women who conceived naturally, researchers found that the number of previous ART cycles emerged as the strongest predictor of postpartum depression. Scientists speculate that certain groups of women may be more vulnerable to mood and anxiety disorders in infertility treatment (Nonacs, *MGH Center for Women's Mental Health*, February 18, 2015). Another study in *Human Reproduction* (Vikstrom, 2017), which comprised 10,412 Swedish women, reported a risk of PPP after IVF treatment. More participants are needed to verify these results.

In 2011 a study was published in *Fertility and Sterility* regarding the psychosocial risks associated with multiple births from ART and those not from ART. The study indicated that mothers with multiples (which can be premature and of low birth weight) encounter more stress than those who underwent ART. (As noted earlier, the two variables often co-occur.) At present researchers conclude that women who conceive using ART are not at significantly elevated risks for postpartum depression, but more research is needed because many women experience elevated levels of anxiety during the pregnancy. The anxiety results from or manifests itself in strained relations with loved ones; persistent feelings of bitterness, anger, pessimism, guilt, or worthlessness; difficulty in concentration; changes in sleep patterns, appetite, or weight; increased use of drugs or alcohol; social isolation; and thoughts about death or suicide.

In March 2015 researchers assessed anger as well as other negative emotions in women who underwent ART (Rosaria et al., *Journal of Maternal-Fetal and Neonatal Medicine*, 2016), and the patients showed quite low levels of tolerance to negative environmental feedback. The study highlights the important role of anger during pregnancy and suggests the need for further studies.

Pregnancy Risks

IVF also has a higher risk of ectopic or tubular pregnancies (2–5 percent compared to 1 percent in traditional pregnancies). A 2013 study in Australia and New Zealand discovered that the lowest risk of ectopic pregnancy was associated with the transfer of a single frozen blastocyst. In June 2015 the European Society for Human Reproduction and Embryology (ESHRE) found a small risk of ectopic pregnancy following ART, but between 2000 and 2012, the risk in the United Kingdom decreased to almost one-half the rate, falling from 20 cases per thousand to 12 (June 2015).

Also, hypertension can complicate pregnancies, according to a May 2016 Greek study in the *Journal of Clinical Hypertension*, and a retrospective study of 596,520 Australian mothers (3.6 percent ART mothers) who gave birth between 2007 and 2011 yielded similar results regarding gestational hypertension and preeclampsia. Researchers attributed the increased risk to multiple pregnancies (Opdahl et al., *Human Reproduction*, July 2015).

A study in *Maternal and Child Health Journal* (Martin, October 2016) found that the odds of developing preeclampsia (an abnormal accumulation of fluids usually toward the end of pregnancy) were increased for deliveries after hyperestrogenic ovarian stimulation. The preeclampsia may in part be related to estrogen associated with the ovarian stimulation.

Morbidity

Researchers also explored trends in severe maternal morbidity or disease after ART and between 2008 and 2012 (Martin et al., *Obstetrics & Gynecology*, January 2016). Researchers found that blood transfusions were the most common severe morbidity for ART and non-ART pregnancies, but singleton pregnancies conceived with ART were at increased risk for more severe maternal morbidity. Fortunately, the rate of morbidity has been decreasing since 2008. In *Fertility and Sterility* (Cromi et al., September 2016) scientists concluded that a history of ART increases the likelihood of needing a hysterectomy to control hemorrhage after birth.

Fetal/Child Risks

At a 2016 meeting of the American Association for the Advancement of Science (AAAS), Pascal Gagneux, an evolutionary biologist from the University of California, San Diego, said children born through IVF could have shorter life spans and poorer health because the healthiest sperm are not always selected during ART (*Daily Telegraph*, February 2016). Some men also are exposed to heavy metals and chemicals that can damage their sperm and cause birth abnormalities.

The past few decades have seen a 200 percent increase in male genital birth defects. Boys have higher incidences of ADHD (attention deficit hyperactivity disorder), learning disabilities, Tourette syndrome, cerebral palsy, and dyslexia. Men exposed to pesticides are more likely to have a child who develops leukemia (Adams, *High Tech Health Newsletter*, November 2013).

On a more positive note, however, the past 20 years have seen a steady improvement in the health outcomes of ART children with fewer babies being born preterm and with low birth weight, stillborn, or dying within the first year of life (ESHRE, 2015).

Risks of Assisted Hatching

Assisted hatching is a procedure usually done on the woman's transplant day and consists of making a hole in the outer shell (zona pellucida) surrounding the embryo. The hole helps the embryo attach to the uterine wall. Risks exist: damage to the embryo, destruction of cells, death of the embryo, and an increased rate of identical twinning.

Risks of Embryo Cryopreservation

Embryo cryopreservation can be done using several different techniques, but all can impact the embryo. Data on fresh versus thawed embryos are lacking, so the difference in the rate of abnormalities will not be known for at least a decade and until large numbers of children are studied.

Preimplantation Genetic Diagnosis

According to Henry T. Greely in *The End of Sex*, preimplantation genetic diagnosis (PGD) has not led to a huge number of miscarriages, stillbirths, or neonatal deaths, but Greely admits that science does not yet have considerable health data on children born following PGD although the procedure has been around for 25 years.

Neurodevelopmental Outcomes

In a review of the literature on neurodevelopmental outcomes in children born after ART (Bay et al., National Agricultural Library, 2013), researchers examined 80 studies. Infants showed no psychomotor deficits, and toddlers reported normal cognitive, behavioral, socioemotional, and psychomotor development. ART children in middle childhood compared favorably with children born after spontaneous conception, and the results for teens are inconclusive at this point.

Birth Defects

More than 3 million children born worldwide because of IVF have been generally healthy although some studies suggest that IVF babies may be at increased risk for birth defects. The risk of birth defects in the normal population is 2–3 percent, but IVF babies carry a reported birth defect rate of 2.6–3.9 percent. The difference is seen usually in singleton males.

In *JAMA Pediatrics* (Boulet, 2016), the authors reported on the frequency of birth defects among live-born infants over a 10-year period. There were 4,553,215 non-ART infants and 64,861 ART infants. The overall risk for birth defects was higher among ART infants, according to the National Health Service of the United Kingdom. Researchers found three factors linked to birth defects: maternal age, smoker or nonsmoker status, and the number of children she had birthed before. Among the smaller group of women who had IVF, the researchers saw no significant link between birth defects and increasing age—neither an increased nor a decreased risk (NHS Choices, States News Service, October 2016).

Imprinting Disorders

Another negative for the ART child involves such imprint disorders as Prader-Willi syndrome, a rare genetic multisystem disorder characterized during infancy by lethargy, diminished muscle tone (hypotonia), feeding difficulties, poor weight gain, and growth hormone deficiency, and Angelman syndrome, another rare genetic neurological disorder characterized by severe developmental delays and learning disabilities; the absence or near absence of speech; an inability to coordinate voluntary movements (ataxia); tremulous, jerky movements of the arms and legs; a distinct behavioral pattern characterized by a happy disposition; and unprovoked episodes of laughter and smiling, often at inappropriate times.

The USDA (U.S. Department of Agriculture) says that children with these syndromes are more likely to be born to parents with fertility problems, but there is no proof at this time of a causal relationship between the diseases and IVF. Two studies concluded that imprinting disorders such as rare genetic disorders like Beckwith-Wiedemann syndrome (an overgrowth disorder usually present at birth and characterized by an increased risk of childhood cancer and certain congenital features) are rare in IVF children.

Risks for Multiples

Geneticists from the Temple University School of Medicine say that while most ART infants are born healthy, some multiples are at higher risk for a range of health problems. An article in the July 2017 issue of *Epigenetics* says that multiples can exhibit lower birth weight or be born prematurely or at risk for development of systemic diseases such as obesity, hypertension, or cardiovascular disease. Researchers say it is not clear whether these variations are a result of ART or due to the parents' struggles with infertility.

Other risks are the double dangers of premature delivery and low birth weight in twins as indicated in a 2010 analysis of 12 studies with a total of 4,385 twins born to women undergoing IVF. Twins and triplets also face an increased risk of cerebral palsy and stillbirth. Some studies in foreign countries connect mental disability to multiple IVF babies (O'Brien, *MarketWatch*, June 2014), and a 2014 paper in the *British Medical Journal* says IVF multiples may have higher blood pressure, higher body fat distribution, and higher glucose levels as well as poorer blood vessel function.

Risks Specific to Male Children

A study by a Brussels professor concluded that of 54 young men (all conceived by ART), all of them had about half the normal sperm concentrate (nearly one-third the sperm count and fewer strong swimmers) of men who conceived naturally. Furthermore, men conceived through intracytoplasmic sperm injection (ICSI) were nearly three times more likely to have sperm concentrations below 15 million per milliliter (the World Health Organization's definition of normal). These findings need to be replicated in a larger group.

Male children conceived through IVF or ICSI often have low birth weights, a higher chance of heart and respiratory issues, and an increased risk for autism or ADHD, according to MedlinePlus (October 2016; see later).

Autism Spectrum Disorder

Children conceived using ICSI were more likely to be diagnosed with autism. Based on a group of 6 million children born in California between 1997 and 2007, these results have led experts to suggest the use of single embryo transfer to minimize the risk of autism spectrum disorder (ASD). The CDC agrees and reports that children conceived using ART were twice as likely to be diagnosed with ASD as children conceived naturally. Evidence also suggests that being born a twin or multiple or born too small increases the risk. About 0.8 percent ART children born as singletons and about 1.2 percent of those born as twins or multiples were diagnosed with ASD. According to the *American Journal of Public Health* (Fountain et al., 2015), researchers speculate that reducing the number of multiple births may also reduce autism rates.

Cognitive Deficits

In 2013 the coauthor of a King's College London Institute of Psychiatry report concluded that IVF involving ICSI (specifically recommended for paternal infertility) is associated with an increased risk of both intellectual disability and autism.

In contrast, a study in Sweden of 99 IVF children (Cederblad et al., *Human Reproduction*, 1996) showed excellent cognitive development, normal behavior, and satisfactory developmental and social adaptation. A more recent study in the December 2015 issue of *European Journal of Developmental Psychology* examined the association between ART and cognitive and social-communication outcomes among preschoolers and found that the ART group of children had higher communicative skills and better motor skills than the spontaneously conceived group.

Cerebral Palsy

An article in *JAMA's Archives of Pediatric Adolescent Medicine* (Hvidtjorn et al., January 2009) reported on nine studies that showed that IVF children had an increased risk of cerebral palsy associated with preterm delivery. Researchers emphasized the serious gaps in knowledge about the long-term outcomes of children born after IVF.

Mental Disorders

A Danish study (Svahn et al., *Human Reproduction*, July 2015) has brought the mental health of ART children to the attention of medical workers. Researchers found an inconsistent and increased risk of hospital admission or outpatient care for mental disorders in 2,412,721 children born to women with fertility problems between 1969 and 2006. Children had a significantly higher risk of mental disorders, including schizophrenia, mood disorders, ADHD, and disorders of psychological development.

Physical Defects

Risks for esophageal atresia (closure of a normal body opening), transesophageal fistula (incorrect communication between two body surfaces or cavities), rectal/large intestine atresia (closure of a normal body opening), and lower limb reduction deformity were higher in ART infants. When organ systems were analyzed separately, the deformities affecting the gastrointestinal tract remained significantly more common. Researchers noted that infertile couples need to be informed of the approximately 30 percent increase in the risk for congenital malformations over the 3–4 percent risk for the general population. A 2013 review of the literature in *Fertility and Sterility* confirmed that ART children are at increased risk of congenital malformations.

Metabolic Abnormalities

Overweight and obese women undergoing ART may be predisposed to giving birth to children with metabolic abnormalities such as reduced glucose consumption, modified amino acid metabolism, and increased levels of triglycerides. These changes in embryonic metabolism may reduce the chances of conception for overweight women. Changes in the embryo during the preimplantation period emphasize the importance of the mother's prepregnancy body weight in optimizing fertility and safeguarding maternal and children's health (Leary et al., *Human Reproduction*, 2015).

Leukemia

A 2016 study in *Pediatrics Week* has both good and bad news for ART children. When researchers analyzed the medical records of more than 1.5 million Norwegian children born from 1984 to 2011 (including 25,782 ART children), the authors found no significant difference between the two groups in the overall risk of developing childhood cancers. However, for specific cancers, ART children were more at risk. For example, they are three times more likely to develop leukemia and have an elevated risk for Hodgkin's lymphoma. In exploring why this diagnosis affected ART children, the authors considered such factors as multiple births, low weight, and infertility experienced by one or both parents (*Pediatrics Week*, April 2016).

Retinoblastoma

Most studies do not report an increased risk of cancer except for retinoblastoma (a treatable eye cancer affecting the retina). In one Netherlands study, five cases were reported following IVF, which is five to seven times more than expected (Medical Centre in Amsterdam, "IVF Babies at Increased Risk for Developing Retinoblastoma," *Transplant News*, March 31, 2003). Also, a report in the *Journal of Family and Reproductive Health* (2013) says ART infants may be born with other ocular problems, among them myopia (nearsightedness), reflex abnormalities, strabismus (abnormal squinting), and poor fixation.

Cardiovascular Issues

Researchers in the June 2014 *Swiss Medical Weekly* pointed out that ART emerges as an important cardiovascular risk factor. This was an unexpected finding in a study of 122 children, 65 of whom were conceived by ART. Young adults (average age of 21) born to mothers who developed preeclampsia during pregnancy face an increased risk of developing hypertension later in life. The 65 ART children also showed marked systemic vascular dysfunction such as narrowed arteries and pulmonary vascular dysfunction.

In 2015 the *European Heart Journal* listed more cardiovascular pathologies among ART youth, including arterial hypertension, cardiac dysfunction, and remodeling in utero as well as insulin resistance. In November 2013, in the *Journal of Clinical Investigation*, researchers showed a relationship between pathological events during fetal development and future cardiovascular risk. Researchers concluded that ART may modify the cardiovascular phenotype (physical characteristics of an organism).

Asthma and Allergies

In a meta-analysis in *BMJ Open* (Nwaru et al., 2016), researchers said recent observations suggest that children conceived through ART may be at increased risk of asthma and allergies.

Mitochondrial Replacement Problems

In 2016 MRT (mitochondrial replacement therapy) debuted because if one female parent's mitochondria does not function properly, it could potentially produce fetal diseases with life-threatening problems. As many as 4,000 children are born with these conditions each year in the United States, and some researchers think that aging eggs correlate with problems in the ART woman's mitochondria. For that reason, physicians sometimes transfer the nuclei of an older woman's egg into the enucleated egg of a healthy young woman or transfer the cytoplasm (including the mitochondria) from a healthy young woman into some of the older woman's eggs.

Dr. John Zhang, a pioneer of MRT, performed this therapy and was able to prevent Leigh syndrome, a fatal neurological disorder, from occurring to the third child of an affected mother. However, a December, 2016 study published in *Nature* suggested that in roughly 15 percent of cases, mitochondrial replacement can fail and allow fatal defects to return or even increase a child's risk for new ailments. The study was conducted at the Oregon Health and Science University in Portland, Oregon.

To prevent this failure, researchers recommend getting a match with a dominating genome so that the defective genome will be completely overwhelmed. Due to these unknowns, a U.S. panel recommended in 2016 that if approved for general use, MRT should be implanted in only male embryos so that the human-altered mitochondrial germ line would not be passed down through the generations.

Chromosomal defects are a main reason for miscarriage and failure to implant in IVF. However, according to ESHRE, the combination of chromosome analysis and mitochondrial assessment may be the most accurate predictor of embryo success in IVF. A study of U.K. and U.S. fertility clinics showed that mitochondrial DNA levels are highly predictive of an embryo's implantation potential. Elevated levels of mitochondrial DNA rarely implant (Fragouli et al., *PLOS Genetics*, June 2015).

Clustered Regularly Interspaced Short Palindromic Repeats

According to Greely, Clustered Regularly Interspaced Short Palindromic Repeats (CRISPR), a gene editing technique that will likely be used in the future, will change the world through its ability to implement fast, cost-effective genome editing. Unlike PGD, a process used to avoid creating sick children, CRISPR will create "designer babies" with enhanced traits. The downside to this is possible mosaicism or potentially dangerous unintended gene editing. Safety trials could eventually eliminate problems, but are the risks worth using it?

Risks from Ultrasound

Scientists have released a cautionary warning to ART patients monitored by ultrasound, especially Doppler. In *Clinical Obstetrics and Gynecology* (Abramowicz, March 2017), the negative susceptibility of the Doppler effect on the oocyte is discussed. Scientists recommend that ultrasound should be used only when medically indicated and only for the shortest possible time at the lowest intensity compatible with accurate diagnosis.

CONCLUSION

Although doctors and scientists know a great deal about the short-term risks of infertility procedures like IVF, they still do not know the results of long-term studies despite these procedures being available for more than 25–30 years. Those risks may be serious or trivial, but until long-term studies take place, scientists and consumers are taking a certain leap of faith at fertility clinics, especially given the possible threats of cancer, autism, and cardiac problems.

Despite the hype of some private clinics, no one can promise a safe, easy ART pregnancy and subsequent birth. Risks exist for both parents and children, ranging from potent hormones that produce mood fluctuations and ovarian chaos to imprinting diseases, mitochondrial misses, and physiological aberrations in fetuses. While this chapter emphasized more of the physical/biological anomalies that can occur in adults and children, the next chapter posits the following question: To what degree do the social and emotional stigmas of ART affect couples, singles, and family members?

PART II

Issues and Controversies

CHAPTER 6

Infertility Stigma

Infertility exists for tens of thousands of people in the United States and other countries. Some people regard infertility as a punishment and use it to blame others or to characterize them as victims or objects of scorn or pity. Such a stigma can mark individuals for disgrace, shame, and even disgust, according to the *International Journal of Gynecology and Obstetrics* (Cook et al., April 2014). Like the stigma of mental illness, the onus of infertility persists despite logic, compassion, fate, and knowledge.

Stigma can take different forms, but the WHO (World Health Organization) says that it usually reduces self-esteem, humiliates, and compromises health. Although Western couples do not experience the extreme social ostracism like third-world countries such as Kenya, where Jackline Mwende's husband chopped off her hands for failing to bear children, they do experience a sense of inadequacy, depression, and personal failure due to the societal emphasis on motherhood, family, and children.

This chapter describes the stigma that infertile people must cope with from friends, family, strangers, and society in general and illustrates how couples deal with it through counseling, e-therapy, and other positive techniques. It also describes stigma's nuanced effects on gender, self-stigmatization, surrogacy, and the workplace.

DIFFERENCES BETWEEN GENDERS

Males

Many infertile couples and individuals resent unwanted questions from friends, family, or strangers. Although women report higher stigma and disclosure than men, men who experience high stigma are associated with lower disclosure (Slade et al., *Human Reproduction*, 2007). Closed-mouthed about their infertility, they often attribute it to impotence or erectile dysfunction, and these feelings contribute to a lower quality of life caused by confusion over their male sexual identity and frustration with the body's perceived deficiency.

Due to these feelings, men often are reticent to get their sperm checked and more apt to avoid mental health services and counseling since few high-profile males and celebrities serve as role models to articulate the problem. Also, research indicates that men who favor powerful masculine attitudes are less apt to seek help.

At five fertility clinics in California, researchers found that 61 percent of men experienced anxiety, but only 24 percent said their fertility center offered them mental health information. The core problem here is anger and anxiety, not clinics unwilling to provide psychosocial help. Negative emotions make men hesitate to get counseling.

Even though researchers correlate sperm DNA damage with everyday stress such as obesity, work, and cell phone use, male patients not only persist in self-blame but also feel a lack of support from family members and health professionals. They report feelings of exclusion from the medical community such as a lack of one-on-one conversations with physicians and unsupportive questions like the following: Have you taken steroids or marijuana? The reason the medical community ignores men is that for doctors, women have the starring roles in Assisted Reproductive Technology (ART) and men are just ancillary. Also, physicians prefer conversing with women because men often come across as more aggressive and less willing to accept medical instructions and protocols.

Although men's emotional responses to infertility have been understudied in comparison to women's, a U.K. paper (Arya et al., *Human Fertility*, 2016) describes how their reactions to ART reinforce the stigma in women. As already noted, men's attitude toward infertility distorts their perceptions of masculinity, and this can interfere with marital relations. Just as physicians tend to cast men as second-class citizens, some men also feel ignored by their relatives, who only seem to seek information from their female partners. Depending on the culture, men can feel desperate about not having children and blame their lack of status on their partners.

Men also suffer by avoiding social gatherings and isolating themselves. After the first year of an infertility diagnosis, studies conclude that men's cognitive deficits include catastrophizing, difficulties in partner communication, and the use of avoidance or religious coping. Their self-image becomes distorted as they feel that their primary goal in life has been denied.

Females

Women experience stigma through marital conflict, sexual problems, and loss of self-esteem. Studies show that depression is the most common symptom, and infertile women grieve as much as individuals with serious medical conditions like cancer and cardiac problems. Women tend to be more emotionally upset than men, especially at times when doctors report the number of eggs harvested, how many were fertilized, and how many were implanted. Women tend to feel personally responsible for the outcomes, and if they are less than ideal, they develop angry and negative feelings and lowered self-esteem. Some women turn against their partners and accuse them of shirking their duty regarding fertility.

Stigma is also exacerbated by disability. Some infertile women identify their infertility as a disability and utilize the Americans with Disabilities Act (ADA) to gain insurance coverage for fertility treatments. In this way they ask society to equate infertility with disability, and although this may be so, the perception imposes a feeling of abnormality on women.

CONFUSING PARENTAL ROLES

The parenting stress placed on women (*Abortion and Art*, summer 2015) communicates that they are bad mothers who somehow rejected their maternal role and put their personal concerns before motherhood. This belief implicitly criticizes women who wish to pursue careers and become pregnant at a later age. Nowadays advances in ART have altered the classic definition of motherhood, and social expectations are struggling to keep up.

Surrogacy Stereotyping

Surrogacy carries both good and bad connotations. Surrogacy challenges the definition of maternity, sometimes regarding surrogates as bad mothers and breeders for hire—empty vessels whose interest in parenting is breeding rather than nurturing young minds. This negative judgment becomes assimilated into women's identity and can cause gender stereotyping that harms women both psychologically and physiologically.

The stress appears less for lesbian couples undergoing IVF than for heterosexual couples. Lesbian couples (and gay fathers) can more easily embrace the experience of motherhood and parenting since they already have overcome one stigma and know that they need medical intervention. Stigma, however, still exists on another level for homosexuals since parents and children do not always resemble each other, and the desire to biologically bond can work against the values of love, trust, and family stability.

The British Warnock Report of 1984 used surrogacy to divide feminists. Women were criticized by other women for deliberately becoming pregnant and giving up the child. Surrogacy does distort the relationship of the mother and child in some ways, which is why Britain banned commercial surrogacy and influenced other countries to do the same.

Popular culture also reinforces stereotypes of commercial surrogates as greedy, uneducated, and dishonest women who do mothering for money and do not parent. This stereotype threatens the genetic-based theory of maternity, but gestational surrogacy rescues it. Although money can be involved in gestational surrogacy, the genetic link is there too.

Another form of surrogate stereotyping is the accusation that women lack the capacity for rational decision making and informed consent. Society questions why a woman would separate pregnancy and maternity and concludes that women either lack reason or use surrogates to make reproduction more convenient. Viewing the surrogate-seeking woman as bad, the public refuses to consider that surrogacy may be necessary for a woman who cannot carry a child to term. In a nonsensical conclusion, the public considers a woman capable of informed consent in all major medical procedures except the decision not to become a mother and instead elect surrogacy or adoption.

The state's stereotyped view is that women will regret their decision, which is why some states impose waiting periods to "protect" women from the consequences of their own decisions. In Michigan, for example, an appeals court rejected a challenge to the state's surrogacy law because it maintained that it needed to prevent the exploitation of women. Many experts say states should not participate in the process of shaming women for their reproductive decisions or denying them their moral rights. (See the "State-by-State Surrogacy Summary" on the Center for Bioethics and Culture website.)

Paradoxically, researchers say families formed through ART tend to be stronger and more highly functioning than naturally conceived ones because the parents are more motivated and gratified to have children. Also, ART can furnish more than two parents or parental figures in children's lives, possibly enriching the emotional environment.

Women Self-Stigmatize

In a 2006 study, 63 percent of women said bearing children is necessary for a woman to have a complete sense of self. Furthermore, findings on two infertility forums hosted by the website Fertile Thoughts (which tracks over 87,000 members) revealed that women avoid conversations related to family or children. Many also admit to selectively disclosing the truth or simply telling lies to avoid uncomfortable discussions.

Belle Boggs, author of *The Art of Waiting: On Fertility, Medicine, and Motherhood* (Graywolf Press, 2016), says she involuntarily started to assume the stereotype of the desperate, uptight infertile woman. She self-stigmatized since her knowledge of the lack of 100 percent success of fertility treatments stressed her everyday life. No wonder that Boggs identifies infertility as "disenfranchised grief," which she defines as grief for a loss that cannot be openly acknowledged, publicly mourned, or socially supported. Women chastise themselves for a loss they keep private and reject the comfort of others.

Women also self-stigmatize their infertility through anger toward their body, guilt and shame for letting their partners down, and denial that they are real women. This attitude hearkens back to Roman times when Juno, the goddess of fertility, gave men permission to swap their wives if they did not bear children. Women sometimes impose a double stigma on themselves: infertility and mental illness. Depressed about their infertility, they develop a neurosis based on their reproductive dysfunction.

Psychosocial Aspects

ART couples must make important decisions, some assisted by fertility specialists and mental health counselors, but other decisions based on individual profiles. For example, many couples on a tight budget can only afford a certain number of IVF cycles. Other contributing factors are age, geographic location, and physical and psychological endurance.

In a June 2016 article on psychosocial interventions in mental health, Liying Ying headed a study of 20 IVF trials that attempted to dispel women's anxiety and negative marital functioning with mind-body interventions such as Eastern body-mind-spirit therapy, cognitive-behavioral therapy, and harp therapy. Although these interventions relieved some stress, they did not relieve the anxiety and depression of IVF patients who were weighing the decision to start or stop IVF. In short, failed IVF treatments increase anxiety, thus emphasizing the importance of post treatment counseling.

Moreover, one of the most difficult fertility-related decisions may be to adopt or not. Qualifying for adoption at different agencies, raising the needed monies, and receiving legal help are probably just as stressful as ART. Experts recommend that before adoption, couples give themselves enough time to grieve for not parenting a child with their own genetic makeup.

ART Children and Stigma

Children who know about their ART origins can feel stigmatized although the ASRM maintains that disclosure to children is usually positive due to benefits. It builds trust among family members, allows families to live honestly rather than in secrecy, fosters bonds between parents and children, avoids unhealthy alliances between those who know and those who do not, eliminates the threat of deception, assures children that it is their right to know about their genetics, and allows parents and children to be honest about their medical histories with healthcare practitioners. Disclosure also encourages children to question and gain understanding, avoids worry about the child finding out by accident, gives parents the opportunity to control the story, and avoids the need for emergency disclosures during medical incidents.

On the other hand, parents may decide not to tell their children because the former are concerned about social stigmatization and teasing. The child's own reaction may preclude disclosure since if the ART children cannot accept an unconventional relationship such as surrogate birth, then their peers certainly will not. Parents also may wish to avoid confusion about identity—for instance, are you really my mother? Sometimes parents have mixed feelings about their gamete donations and feel ART is a less healthy form of family building.

Pronatalism versus Childless

Pronatalism expresses the belief that a woman's social value is linked to her production of biological children. For some of the 5 million infertile women in the United States, bearing a child is impossible, and their experiences in a pronatalist society have been given little attention. Interviews with 32 infertile participants revealed that women usually experienced the pronatalist ideology through insensitive comments, questions, and unsolicited advice. Infertile women usually responded by immersing themselves in their work, leisure activities, or support groups.

Pronatalism, however, extends beyond its human population. Social controls of pronatalism are used to aid survival and perpetuate power in established institutions like the government, the church, and business. Governments encourage births so that tax bases can grow, churches and other houses of worship want their congregants to cherish childbirth to ensure their longevity as members, and businesses reap the rewards of a pro-parenthood society through healthy economic growth in products and services. Advertisers use the social values of pregnancy and parenting as sales and marketing tools. Sentimentalized images of children are juxtaposed with a variety of products—for instance, vacations, cereals, cars, and insurance. Madison Avenue uses "family" to sell things whether the product is designed for that or not. How many times have we flipped through magazine ads where cute babies are selling merchandise like carpeting or toilet paper?

The entertainment media also revel in pronatalistic themed programs. *Sesame Street* and animated movies enrapture adults and children alike, and where else but in a child-centric society would television shows flourish like *19 Kids and Counting* featuring the Duggars, *Kate Plus Eight*, *Raising Sextuplets*, and *Table for 12*.

Differing Opinions

ART procedures often trigger controversies and conflicts. Friends and family sometimes do not agree with the couple's decision, and if they voice those opinions, relationships can suffer. Too often friends and family blunder when conversing about babies, and women and their partners experience feelings of loss and criticism as well as resentment of their "fishbowl" existence.

According to the national association RESOLVE, family and friends can best be emotionally supportive by acknowledging the infertility and asking how things are going or how a friend is feeling. Also, they can ask friends or loved ones to share any information on infertility. Everyone must be realistic about the pain that accompanies infertility so that honesty pervades the relationships. If couples feel overwhelmed, they should say so and ask for understanding, patience, and guidance. The main function friends can play is as good listeners. Couples need to share their grief and vent their negative feelings, and they need trustworthy sounding boards to help them move on to more positive perspectives.

Friends also need to accept different ways of coping—for example, couples' refusals to attend potentially uncomfortable events such as baby showers, christenings, and family reunions. Partners need to know that their friends respect them and realize they are multifaceted people in which infertility plays only one part. Friends need to respect other couples' desires for a child even if they do not agree with the method of attaining that goal.

IVF Stigma on Parenting

IVF couples aim to be perfect parents, and parenting itself is so loaded with societal pressures to excel that the incentive can be even greater for IVF parents. The assumption is that since the couples actively sought parenthood, they should be obligated not to be merely good at nurturing but great. Journalists describe this as "aggressive cultivation." This phenomenon has taken the pronatalist norm to new heights because parents often use their children as a tool for status, achievement, and recognition.

However, parents of IVF babies may have a more difficult transition to parenthood than other parents, one reason being they are usually older and have less support from their own parents or peers who had children years before them. Also, while getting fertility treatment, IVF couples may have avoided babies and children for psychological protection, and this may have affected not only their parenting skills but also their realistic expectations of the demands of babies and young children.

Furthermore, due to IVF couples' steady dependence on medical experts guiding them through the ART process, they may rely more on expert models of parenting than on common sense. They may cope with parenting challenges by turning to celebrity mavens rather than trusting their own intuition (Bailey, June 2016). The results of the Hjelmstedt paper (Hjelmstedt et al., 2004), for instance, implied that IVF parents may benefit from counseling since half of them believe that they experienced parenthood differently from other parents. They had stronger feelings toward their infants, a higher tolerance for the difficulties of raising a child, and increased worry. Some parents concern themselves about their child's reactions to IVF treatments and want to guarantee a positive slant. Other parents felt that keeping mementos of the IVF period was proof of the child's uniqueness and would make the child feel appreciated and desired.

Stigma: Child as Commodity

Eighteenth-century philosopher Immanuel Kant uses the term "commodity" in the context of reproduction to indicate a child regarded as a purchase. Nowadays that so-called commodity can be created via IVF, intracytoplasmic sperm injection (ICSI), artificial insemination (AI), or other ART, but its origins stem from a medical procedure that deals in supply and demand. The overwhelming media attention to IVF may result in parents regarding their child as a possession instead of a gift. Kant says this attitude violates the child's human dignity and autonomy. Kant's ethical theory revolves around the "golden rules" of morality. One such moral imperative is never to use someone as a mere means; actions must treat the child as a desirable end and never as just a means. Thus, creating a "savior sibling" (see Chapter 10) simply as a source of fetal stem cells for healing or curing another child would be morally wrong, according to Kant. The "savior" must be created because of its own intrinsic value and preciousness.

Commodification must be carefully avoided especially considering emerging reproductive technologies such as preimplantation genetic diagnosis (PGD), clustered regularly interspaced short palindromic repeats (CRISPR), and mitochondrial replacement therapy (MRT; see further information in Chapters 5 and 9). These processes have the potential to treat babies as commodities, permitting parents not only to screen for genetic diseases but also to select for gender and other physical characteristics. The fear is that this could lead to the commercialization of entire bodies and organs and become a crass method of reproduction like human reproductive cloning.

Another argument against IVF and other similar procedures is that it is exploitative—for example, selling gametes for hundreds of dollars. This could deprive the child of a known genetic parentage.

DESTIGMATIZING INFERTILITY AND ART

To minimize the conflicts surrounding infertility, individuals should seek out advocacy groups like the American Pregnancy Organization, Society for Assisted Reproductive Technology (SART), American Society for Reproductive Medicine (ASRM), and RESOLVE. Their resources, especially the online forums, can reduce fear and anxiety and give confidence to fertility treatments. Also, counseling paves the way for feelings based on logic and compassionate understanding rather than negativity.

E-Therapy

E-therapy is fast becoming beneficial for people grappling with significant issues such as IVF or adoption. It is convenient and can link people to educational materials. According to the website Metanoia, which links to mental health resources, 60 percent of 450 patients who tried e-therapy found it very helpful, 32 percent found it somewhat helpful, and 8 percent did not find it helpful at all.

In fertility care, personalizing an e-therapy program according to the patients' risk profile can reduce psychological distress and treat current symptoms of anxiety and depression. However, individuals should also seek professional one-on-one help when exhibiting symptoms like bitterness, lack of motivation, difficulty maintaining relationships, and changes in appetite or sleeping patterns.

Another technique to reduce negative psychological consequences, especially in men, are online discussion boards. Findings by Jeremie Richard et al. (*American Journal of Men's Health*, 2016) on 199 users chatting on two boards showed that infertile men can expand their social network while acquiring support from people with similar experiences. Four types of social support (appraisal, emotional, informational, and instrumental) were used as strategies, but appraisal was used most often. Five themes also were identified to convey emotional feedback: normalization of the emotional roller coaster; personal experience; disappointment in self and fear that wife holds male responsible; isolation encountered from wives, family, friends, and coworkers; and the connectedness of men's experiences of fertility. The authors concluded that an available online peer support network facilitated men's connectedness regarding fertility problems through a secure, accessible, and anonymous media.

Counseling and Support Groups

According to the ASRM, infertility is as grief provoking as the death of a family member, separation, or divorce. That is why licensed clinical social workers have helped couples for years, providing counseling and third-party reproduction insights on using a donor egg, sperm, embryo, or surrogate. A professional evaluates all parties to make sure no psychological issues can interfere, develops counseling recommendations, and helps couples clarify their expectations and analyze potential decisions. Referrals for short-term counseling often work the best if they begin before the patient starts infertility treatments. Health experts can then provide information on how to manage fatigue, reduce stress and anxiety, and improve communication.

Counseling helps people understand that feelings of anger and sadness are normal, and blaming is harmful. They learn that communicating with partners and creating intimacy helps everyone feel more in control, that continuing with hobbies and attending cultural and social events provides balance, that pampering with massages or pedicures helps the patient feel special, and that experimenting with prayer and meditation can achieve calmness.

Expressive Writing

Sometimes expressive writing can reduce distress by helping people to cope with unpleasant experiences, minimize depressive symptoms, and improve the physical condition of ART patients. In a study described in *Human Reproduction* (December 2016), researcher Yoon Frederiksen concluded that expressive writing intervention (EWI) significantly reduced depressive symptoms but not anxiety and infertility-related distress. He then used EWI to encourage the expression of feelings about infertility that are sometimes perceived as socially unacceptable. The trial participants consisted of 295 men and women who were asked to write about their daily lives for 20 minutes three times during the period between IVF and pregnancy. Half the participants were asked to write about their emotional challenges, and the others, a control group, were asked to write about ordinary daily activities. The results were surprising: the method improved the depressive symptoms in women, but men became more stressed. Many women also can take advantage of online blogging at sites like https://weforgotthe sperm.com/ and https://thegreatpuddingclubhunt.com/.

ART Stigma in the Workplace

At least one in eight couples struggles with infertility stigma silently in the workplace, according to a survey of 1,000 adults in March 2017 by Come Recommended. The half of respondents who discussed their infertility at work felt supported in the workplace, but the other half who chose not to bring up their infertility reported a poor workplace experience. They quit their jobs, looked for new ones, or continued working even though they were unhappy. Support was so important to them that they prioritized it above work-life balance, a good job, wellness initiatives, salary, or perks. Although every company cannot afford fertility benefits such as egg freezing or IVF cycles, some employers might consider a fertility coach or paid medical leave that includes time off for infertility appointments and treatments for free or discounted services such as acupuncture or yoga.

Stressed-out employees feel more supported if they can talk about fertility empathetically with the human resources department, their direct supervisor, or coworkers. Otherwise their colleagues may make false assumptions (e.g., that their infertility is a lifestyle choice) or unintentionally isolate the employee. Colleagues should not ask questions such as are you planning to have kids, and they should not try to minimize the problem by saying, don't worry about it or try to solve it by recommending different fertilization methods. Also, they should not gossip but should respect their colleague's privacy.

CONCLUSION

The stigma accompanying ART is not easy to ignore, especially the surrogate stigma, with its long reputation of exploiting women for payment and separating pregnancy from maternity. Also, disclosure of infertility in a pronatalist culture can be difficult, especially when gender stereotyping demeans women for not being mothers and regards married childless men as immature weaklings lacking the machismo to impregnate their wives.

IVF is far from painless, inexpensive, or natural. It differs radically from the average woman's spontaneous conception, and decisions arise around every corner. Sometimes couples need counseling help or e-therapy to help them manage their finances, their emotions, and their options such as surrogacy and adoption. Some couples pressure themselves by feeling that their investment of time and energy in ART should make them super parents, and something is wrong with them if they are just average.

Experts suggest techniques to relieve the stigma of ART, but these methods do not always work. Confiding to people at work may help some employees, but others may benefit more from speaking to friends and relatives or keeping the medical protocol a secret while expressing emotions in a personal journal.

Psychosocial pressures can impact couples in different ways, but no one gets off easy, and counseling plays a heavy role in infertility therapy. The next chapter discusses other cultural challenges for ART couples: religion and race. These factors can stir up emotions in a variety of contexts and complicate decision making even more.

CHAPTER 7

ART Challenges for Religion and Race

Designer babies are still wishful thinking, and even if Assisted Reproductive Technology (ART) and preimplantation genetic diagnosis (PGD) could guarantee certain personality and character traits, many parents would not want to act against their theological beliefs. Although some people do not care what their religion dictates (or, for that matter, do not consider themselves members of any one religion), many adults adhere to a spiritual belief and feel they must abide by the teachings of the Torah, the Koran, the Bible, or some other religious tract.

This chapter not only examines the contradictions between certain religious values and ART but also reveals the racism in the United States that compromises ART's accessibility to blacks. Primarily targeted to Caucasians due to economic realities, ART should have global appeal to couples of all races seeking fertility treatments. However, blacks in the United States have not embraced IVF in high numbers. Why this is so is discussed later in this chapter.

ART AND HELP SEEKING IN THE UNITED STATES

The 2013 Pew Research Center's Religion & Public Life Project indicates that there are only modest differences in opinions about the moral acceptability of IVF among religious groups. Forty-six percent of Americans among a national sample of 4,006 adults say they do not consider IVF to be a moral issue. Morality or ethical concerns that lead to help seeking are associated with greater religiosity, which is defined as regular attendance at a church, temple, or mosque, according to a 2010 study of 2,183 infertile women in the United States.

Although some religious women seek medical help or help from alternative healers, other women base their help seeking on mediating variables such as a greater belief in the importance of motherhood and adoption (*Social Science Medicine*, August 2010). That may be because religion and pronatalism go hand in hand, and women are encouraged to pursue infertility health issues because religions in general approve of healthy lifestyle habits, provide social support, bolster self-esteem and self-efficacy, and provide a structure for interpreting life events.

The above study also incorporated racial attitudes and concluded that black, Hispanic, and Asian women express greater ethical concerns about infertility treatment than white women, and these concerns were positively associated with higher levels of religious attendance. Black and Hispanic women scored lower on the importance of motherhood, which may help explain their worse IVF outcomes and the fact that only 8 percent of black women and 8 percent of Latinas between the ages 25 and 44 sought medical help compared to 15 percent of white women. However, the interrelationship between ethnicity and help seeking is complex and requires more research.

While all religions support pronatalism, they differ in how they interpret the ethics of fertility treatments.

Judaism and ART

Broadly speaking, Jews allow ART because their liturgy encourages them to bear children: "Be fruitful and multiply, fill the earth and subdue it" (Gen. 1:28) proclaims the Bible. Jews are instructed to improve the world and ensure that humanity does not become extinct.

However, the three Jewish sects—Orthodox, Conservative, and Reformed—vary in their degrees of acceptance of ART. PGD is allowed by all three divisions because, according to theological writings, the soul does not enter the body until after 40 days and PGD prevents serious genetic diseases such as Tay-Sachs.

Selective reduction (abortion of embryos) is considered acceptable since it enhances the possibility of life as determined by doctors; therapeutic cloning (the production of embryonic stem cells for use in replacing or repairing damaged tissues or organs) is also acceptable as well as life-saving treatments such as stem cell and cellular replacement therapy.

The main controversy within the Jewish faith relates to third-party reproduction such as adopting gametes. While Conservative and Reform Jews accept the use of anonymous sperm, most Orthodox rabbis reject this. Orthodox clergy also contend that the spilling of the seed is forbidden, and consequently, the husband may not ejaculate (masturbate) to provide a specimen. Some Orthodox rabbis, however, permit nonmedicated condoms to collect sperm, and other more liberal rabbis permit ejaculation if the intention is to enhance procreation.

The Rabbinical Assembly's Committee on Jewish Law and Standards recommends that Conservative Jews use the following protocol: First use artificial insemination (AI) with sperm from the husband or donor and then try IVF as a fallback. Egg donation is the next option and surrogacy last of all. Up to three embryos may be transferred at once for implantation, and embryos may be frozen.

Sperm cryopreservation is controversial when used outside the boundaries of marriage since artificial insemination by donor is prohibited in Judaism because Jewish law believes that getting pregnant by donor sperm implies a series of problems related to parentage and identity. Also, most rabbis do not allow egg or embryo donation because if the genetic mother is not Jewish, the child cannot be considered Jewish. Gender selection is allowed but only for couples who have at least four children of the same sex (family gender balancing).

When an exception is made, rabbis usually prefer a non-Jewish sperm donor since Jewishness is conveyed through the mother's line. AI also is recommended in situations where the husband suffers from anatomical defects of the penis or from severe psychological impotence. It is also used when the husband has a low sperm count.

While most rabbis do not accept surrogacy due to the surrogate receiving economic compensation, those who do allow surrogacy prefer the use of single Jewish women. In Portland, Oregon, Rabbi Michael Cahana helps gay men acquire children from a surrogate mother who is not Jewish. He "converts" the babies later by having the father dip the babies underwater in a mikveh (spa-like arrangement). Since posthumous donation is not part of a marriage, it is not permissible in more conservative denominations. Since children are considered a blessing, Jewish law states that husband and wife should follow the command of having at least two children—through normal conception, ART, or adoption.

ROMAN CATHOLICISM AND ART

USA Network reports that Catholics object to using sperm or egg donors. All forms of ART, including intrauterine insemination (IUI), IVF, intracytoplasmic sperm injection (ICSI), and surrogate motherhood, are forbidden, but IUI can be accepted if the semen is collected by sexual intercourse. AID (artificial insemination by donor) is forbidden because it involves a third party. The Roman Catholic Church, which strongly supports the protection of human life from conception, disapproves of cryopreservation, abortion (selective reduction), and research on embryos.

But some Catholics regard embryo adoption as prenatal adoption—an alternative that leads to the possibility of giving spare embryos the chance to live. According to some Catholics, unused embryos are full-fledged human beings despite being conceived in a morally unacceptable way. For devout Catholics every fertilization process that does not take place through sexual acts in marriage translates into a nonhuman way of

conceiving a child. Catholics are opposed to surrogacy because the conceived baby does not carry the genetic material of both parents.

Infertile couples who are not strict adherents to the faith often utilize
some reproductive options. Aggressive ovulation induction is an example.
Catholic doctrine allows fertility drugs, and if the eggs are combined with
intercourse rather than IUI, this technique is considered moral.

Some Catholics also recognize gamete intrafallopian transfer (GIFT) as
morally acceptable. Eggs are retrieved laparoscopically, combined with
sperm, and reimplanted into the fallopian tube. This fulfills the requirements of intracorporeal (within the body) fertilization, and some Catholic
patients have intercourse timed to this fertility procedure to allow for the
possibility that the sperm that fertilizes the egg may have been conjugally
ejaculated. The Catholic Church opposes PGD—despite critics touting the
major medical benefits PGD provides—based on the ethical grounds that
PGD can lead to the destruction of embryos that the church maintains
are equal to full-fledged persons.

PROTESTANTISM AND ART

Christian bioethicists agree that most forms of surrogacy are theologically
and morally problematic due to the exploitation of women, the "selling" or
commodification of children, the violation of the marital bond, and the use
of embryo-destructive technology. Also, some Christians maintain that surrogacy can confuse the child's identity and disrupt the natural links between
marriage, conception, gestation, birth, and parenting. Adults involved in surrogacy must not behave as though they alone are affected; the concepts of
autonomy and reproductive freedom are also rights of the child.

Protestant denominations vary in their beliefs about IVF and do not
have one set of ethical guidelines as the Catholic Church does. Those
who support IVF limit its use to married couples. All embryos must be
replaced into the uterus—selective reduction is not allowed, but embryo
adoption is. For instance, embryo adoption can be handled through a
U.S. project known as "Snowflakes." A division of Nightlight Christian
Adoptions, Snowflakes has accumulated embryos from 1,200 families,
and 500 families have adopted them.

The Anglican church does not offer a moral status to the embryo
and believes this can only be conferred on an individual with a well-
established personality. Thus, it allows IVF and embryo transfer, enabling
the doctors to use sperm obtained after masturbation. The church has
recently accepted gamete donation by third parties although individuals
may decide not to use it.

The Church of England does not approve of ART for single women and
gay couples, especially surrogacy. Church officials stated in 2012 that
bringing the care of an adoptive home to a needy child is a wholly

different circumstance from using IVF technology for surrogacy. This equates to having a child by design who will never have a father (or mother in the case of gay men commissioning a child by surrogacy).

The Eastern (Greek) Orthodox Church allows the medical and surgical treatment of infertility including using the husband's sperm in IUI. It does not accept IVF and other ART procedures such as surrogate motherhood, donor insemination, and embryo donation. The church suggests adoption as an alternative. If this is not feasible, then the church approves fertilization techniques that do not involve surplus embryos or include any form of donation or embryo destruction. The church also accepts the use of only the parents' gametes and the fertilization of as many embryos as will be implanted.

The Coptic Orthodox Church is more lenient than other Eastern Orthodox churches. IVF is accepted if the oocyte and sperm are taken from the parents and fertilization occurs in vitro with no doubt about gamete mixing. Embryo transfer must take place in the mother, who is the source of the oocytes. AI with the husband's sperm is also accepted, but gamete donation is not.

Other Christian sects (except for Christian Science) have more liberal attitudes. They accept IVF with spouses' gametes and no embryo wastage; however, gamete donation is forbidden. The above prohibitions refer to Baptist, Methodist, Lutheran, Mormons, Presbyterian, Episcopal, United Church of Christ, Jehovah's Witnesses, Seventh-day Adventists, and Mennonites. Mormons also strongly discourage the use of surrogate parents, but the Church of Jesus Christ of Latter-day Saints believes this decision should ultimately be left to the husband and wife.

The Christian Science Church does not accept IVF due to the use of medication and surgical techniques (laparoscopic procedures) but leaves the final decision to individual couples. It also opposes gamete donation and surrogacy but has no objection to using AI with the husband's sperm.

ISLAM AND ART

Islam is based on four principles: Any act is permitted unless the Koran prohibits it; any act should produce no harm and should not be done under harassment. Necessity permits the prohibited, and if two necessary acts are harmful, one should choose the one leading to the least harm. Islam also emphasizes the importance of marriage, family, and procreation, but adoption in the legal sense is not permitted (although raising or "sponsoring" a child not genetically related to oneself is allowed).

SUNNI (ISLAM) AND ART

All forms of ART are allowed if the sperm and oocyte are those of the husband and his wife and the embryo is placed into the wife's uterus during an existing marriage contract. A third party cannot be involved, thus excluding the possibility of sperm and egg donation as well as surrogacy.

Cryopreservation of sperm, eggs, and embryos is allowed. According to the Koran, the soul enters the fetus after 120 days, after which it cannot be destroyed. Thus, selective reduction is allowed if the pregnancy is failing or the mother's life is in jeopardy.

Pregnancy after menopause is allowed when using cryopreserved oocytes of the same woman in an existing marriage. Therapeutic cloning (the production of embryonic stem cells for use in replacing or repairing damaged tissues or organs) for regenerative medicine is also allowed, but reproductive cloning is prohibited. Somatic gene therapy is allowed, but germ line gene therapy is still debated. (Somatic cell gene therapy changes, fixes, or replaces genes in just one person, and the changes are not passed on to that person's offspring, but germ line gene therapy makes permanent changes in the sperm or egg of an individual.)

Surrogacy is not permitted, but the use of PGD to avoid genetic diseases is allowed and considered better than prenatal diagnosis and abortion. PGD sperm selection techniques for sex preselection is not allowed for the first child, but a recent ruling allows PGD for fair balancing if the couple already has two children of the same gender.

Shi'a (Islam) and ART

The Shi'a principles and practices are similar to those of the Sunni except for one difference: Shias allow gamete donation—thus the child of the egg donor has the right to inherit from his or her biological mother. The baby born of sperm donation will follow the name of the infertile father rather than the sperm donor, and, as with egg donation, the donor child can only inherit from his or her biological father since the infertile father is considered to be an adoptive father. Yale professor and religious specialist Marcia C. Inhorn says an increasing number of Muslims practicing Shiite Islam use donors, especially egg donors.

Gestational surrogacy is also accepted. Shi'a Muslims are encouraged to practice a certain form of individual religious reasoning that has led to several disagreements about the permissibility and prohibition of certain ART strategies.

A summary follows:

a. Artificial insemination with the husband's semen is allowed, and the resulting child is the legal offspring.
b. In a medical necessity, the IVF of an egg from the wife with the sperm of her husband can result in a fertilized embryo that is transferred to the wife.
c. No third-party participation for sperm, eggs, embryos, or uterus is allowed.

d. Adoption is not allowed.
e. Posthumous conception is not allowed.
f. Cryopreservation is allowed and is the property of the couple alone.
g. Fetal reduction is only allowed if multiple pregnancies endanger the other embryos or the health of the mother.
h. No traditional surrogacy is allowed, only gestational.
i. Establishment of sperm or egg banks is forbidden.
j. A qualified physician is the only person who can practice these procedures.

HINDUISM AND ART

Because Hinduism puts great importance on childbearing, it is very liberal, agreeing with most ART principles but insisting that the oocyte and the sperm come from a married couple. Hinduism accepts sperm donations, but the donor must be a close relative of the infertile husband. Also, abortion is allowed as is postmortem sperm donation, gene selection, and adoption. Since lineage does not depend on a genetic tie, women who can afford ART may solicit it. This liberal attitude has made India an important destination for reproductive tourism, and many couples travel there for ART and surrogacy, including members of the LGBT communities.

BUDDHISM AND ART

Like Hinduism, Buddhism is liberal and uses "harm" as the yardstick against which a person should measure any action. It allows IVF without restricting its access to married couples, and sperm donation is permitted. A child conceived from donated genetic material has the right to meet his or her genetic parents as he or she reaches maturity. Also allowed are ICSI, PGD, and surrogacy. Since it is impossible for humans to determine whether a soul is present in a specific embryo, people should err on the side of caution and treat all leftover embryos as though they contain a soul. Embryos should not be harmed, so disposing of leftover embryos at the end of an IVF cycle can be ethically problematic. Buddhist principles seem to require fertilizing only as many eggs as will be implanted.

FOLK CULTURES AND OTHER RELIGIONS

More than 400 million people practice folk or traditional religions, including African, Chinese, Native American, and Australian aboriginal. The practice of IUI, IVF, ICSI, cryopreservation, and PGD are allowed in China (where Confucianism, Taoism, and Buddhism are practiced). The following procedures are prohibited: sex selection without medical reasons, surrogate motherhood, embryo donation, gamete donation, and human reproductive cloning. Shintoism is a popular faith in Japan, where the law allows IUI, IVF, and ICSI. Donor insemination is also permitted in Shintoism, but if both partners are infected with HIV, oocyte donation and surrogacy are prohibited as is IVF.

WEIGHING THE IMPORTANCE OF RELIGION WHEN CONSIDERING ART

According to Arthur L. Greil, sociology professor at Alfred University in New York, many infertile couples do not heed religious advice. Studies have found high levels of public support for ART—sometimes as high as 90 percent for IVF and 20–60 percent for AID (artificial insemination by donor), and surrogacy. A *New York Times* journalist found that while Roman Catholics were upset over the release of the Vatican instructions, they did not allow these instructions to influence their choice of treatment. Greil said his interviews with infertile couples indicate that such indifference to religious objections is widely shared. If couples reject treatment, it is usually not because the next step was morally repugnant, but rather because the couple was tired of the process, could not afford the cost, or saw adoption as a faster means of realizing their goal.

RACISM IN ART

Between 2005 and 2011, a survey revealed that 80 percent of respondents who froze their eggs at New York University were white. Only 4 percent were black. Desiree McCarthy-Keith, a fertility specialist in Atlanta, Georgia, said black women have been left out of the egg freezing loop and might not even know about egg freezing even though SART predicts that by 2018 76,000 women will freeze their eggs. The reason for this expected increase in egg freezing is that women trust the technology because the survival rate for eggs is near 90 percent and over 95 percent for embryos.

Ironically, the rate of infertility is nearly twice as likely to affect blacks as it does whites. Among black women, 11.5 percent are reporting fertility struggles, compared to 7 percent of white women. McCarthy-Keith of Georgia Reproductive Specialists reports that black women are also less likely to pursue fertility treatments. In the past the problem of infertility in minority women was rarely addressed, and most marketing campaigns of infertility awareness were not directed toward blacks. This omission resulted in their lack of awareness about infertility, evaluation, and treatment. The high cost of ART can also limit families from poorer ethnic and minority backgrounds. Some anthropologists of reproduction speculate that there is a scholarly tacit attitude that the poor are unworthy of infertility treatments.

Although fertility struggles among African Americans are less likely to be treated by IVF, it is not completely unheard of. At times, the embryos created for an African American couple through IVF are more than what the couple can use for their own family building. Embryos can then be donated to another black couple who may desire to build their family through embryo adoption. Stacey Edwards-Dunn, who created the nonprofit Fertility for Colored Girls, calls infertility in the black community "The Silent Giant." She had eight rounds of IVF before her daughter was born.

Monica Simpson, executive director of SisterSong, a reproductive justice organization for minority women, stated that black women bear a stigma in various reproductive areas. They are criticized for having too many babies they cannot afford, for being too picky and not finding a man, for having multiple children, and for the decision to use IVF heterosexually or in a lesbian relationship. Simpson says a real divide exists between white and black women. She hopes the fertility industry will realize their narrowness and that black women will accept egg freezing as not just an intended treatment for their wealthier white peers.

According to Miriam Zoll's book *Cracked Open: Liberty, Fertility, and the Pursuit of High-Tech Babies*, the fertility clinics mainly cater to white upper-class couples and singles who can afford to pay despite the lack of insurance.

Studies of black women participating in ART are confusing and contradictory at best. In *Fertility and Sterility* (Seifer et al., November 2008), the researchers concluded that black women, who represented 7.8 percent of married reproductive-age women in the United States, were underrepresented among IVF recipients. For example, after controlling for increased tubal and uterine factor infertility among African Americans, black women were an independent risk factor for not achieving a live birth. In a more recent study in *Fertility and Sterility* (Blake et al., September 2016), researchers evaluated the impact of race on live birth rates in recipients of donor oocytes and found that uterine factors may contribute to worse outcomes in black women.

In a literature review in the *American Journal of Obstetrics & Gynecology* (February 2016), Leigh A. Humphries from the Beth Israel Deaconess Medical Center in Boston, Massachusetts, identified 24 IVF studies. Black, Hispanic, and Asian women had lower clinical pregnancy rates and/or live birth rates after IVF was compared with white women. Although current evidence points to race and ethnicity (especially the black race), as strong predictors of poorer outcomes after IVF, the results are also affected by such limitations as sample size and selection bias. In other words, researchers are unsure just why race affects ART rates. Further studies are needed to better understand the pervasiveness of racial disparities in IVF outcomes.

Dorothy Roberts in Chapter 6 of *Killing the Black Body: Race, Reproduction and the Meaning of Liberty* (Pantheon, 1997) describes how women of color have historically experienced "reproductive punishment" or "reproductive oppression" as defined by ACRJ (Asian Communities for Reproductive Justice). (ACRJ is a founding member of the SisterSong Women of Color Reproductive Health Collective, the largest national multiethnic reproductive justice collective.) Dorothy Roberts's research indicates that reproductive oppression is a means of selectively controlling the destiny of entire communities through rainbow women populations. One channel of control is through the expense of IVF, which is beyond the affordability range of most black women. Only about one-third of black couples experiencing infertility seek medical treatment, and only 10–15 percent of infertile couples seeking treatment use ART procedures like IVF. Blacks make up a disproportionate number of infertile people who avoid reproductive technologies while white women who seek treatment for fertility are twice as likely to undergo high-tech treatments as black women.

Only 12.8 percent of black women in the latest national survey used specialized infertility services such as drugs, AI, tubal surgery, or IVF compared with 27.2 percent of white women. Even black couples who can afford the amenities of a middle-class lifestyle refrain from turning to high-tech fertility services.

The reason? It is hard for black women to trust the medical establishment when their race sometimes determines their diagnosis of infertility. For example, doctors attribute endometriosis mainly to white women, but most gynecology textbooks lead doctors to diagnose black women as infertile due to pelvic inflammatory disease (which they treat with sterilization) or fibroids rather than endometriosis. In 1976, however, doctors found that over 20 percent of black patients diagnosed with pelvic inflammatory disease suffered from endometriosis.

CONCLUSION

Despite the anti-ART injunctions of some religions, couples are not shying away from high-tech procedures on religious grounds. Perhaps due to the desire of churches and temples to retain members of different faiths, theological beliefs are becoming more liberal and responsive to their congregants. Furthermore, practical concerns overshadow ethical precepts and encourage a Judeo-Christian pragmatic morality (Magelssen et al., *Ethics & Medicine*, 2015). Practicing Catholics, however, are still on the lower end of the ART permissiveness scale.

Race is more influential with respect to ART than religion is. Black females do not have much faith in ART, but younger white adults feel confident that their infertility will yield to ART procedures. Cryopreservation is their fallback technique for conception. On the other hand, many of their black counterparts do not trust the medical establishment and their fertility treatments.

In Chapter 8 religion takes a back seat to ethics and the behavioral intentions of would-be parents. The essential question is the following: Should parents make decisions that may fall outside of acceptable ethical standards and what happens when they do?

ART Ethics Affecting Parents

To engineer ethical Assisted Reproductive Technology (ART) births, couples must apply religious and philosophical beliefs, social and cultural mores, and attitudes of reproductive responsibility, human rights, and fairness. The conflicts between what intended parents want and what is beneficial for parent, child, and society complicate the ethics of ART, but most couples overcome these hurdles with the help of counselors, clergy, and common sense. They apply the four commonly accepted pillars of healthcare ethics regarding reproductive technology: respect for autonomy, nonmaleficence, beneficence, and justice.

This chapter discusses these four pillars of healthcare ethics in terms of 10 ART-related parental areas: relative's gametes; surrogacy; the number of IVF cycles; nonregulation; elective single embryo transfer (eSET); populations of singles, HIV patients, and LGBTs; posthumous ART; mitochondria donation; human cloning; and informed consent.

THE FOUR PILLARS

According to the Medical Ethics 101 class at Stanford University, autonomy requires that the patient must be free of coercion regarding healthcare decision making. The patient must understand all the risks and benefits and the likelihood of success. Justice, the second pillar, requires that procedures be fair to all those involved and that the burdens and benefits of new or experimental treatments be distributed equally among all groups in society. The healthcare provider must consider the fair distribution of scarce resources; competing needs, rights, and obligations; and potential conflicts with established legislation. Beneficence, the third pillar, translates to the need for the procedure's intent to benefit the patient, and nonmaleficence requires that a procedure not harm the patient or society physically or emotionally.

ETHICS OF USING RELATIVES' GAMETES

Couples are increasingly turning to relatives, especially siblings, for gamete donations. A 2016 article by *Glamour* editor Liz Brody informs readers that 5–10 percent of women receive donor eggs from siblings. Why is family fertility help becoming a trend? For one thing, the genetic link is there—a sibling's genotype is the closest thing to having your own biological child. It also diminishes the risk of genetic or sexually transmitted infections and is cheaper since the donor probably will not charge his or her sibling. Also, it speeds up the ART process, and the couple gains much more information on the donor than if the gamete came from an anonymous source. Given all these advantages, is this sibling arrangement ethical?

Although some experts warn against potentially incestuous relationships, laws banning intercourse and marriage between siblings permit donor gametes because no actual sexual relations or marriages occur. However, the Centre for Family Research at the University of Cambridge, United Kingdom, regards cross-generational gamete donation (such as daughter to mother) as unethical presumably because coercion (and not autonomy) may take place. Unusual reproductive links like this can create familial tensions. A greater ethical problem, though, is that donors might blame themselves if a miscarriage occurs, or the child has a genetic or birth defect. On the other hand, donations from relatives can build feelings of family solidarity. Sibling donation is especially positive for gay couples, who usually do not have an infertility problem but are routinely recommended for IVF. In this way they can save money.

How do adults cope emotionally with relatives' donations? A 2016 study (Wyverkens) in the *Journal of Reproductive and Infant Psychology* performed an interpretative phenomenological analysis, and 10 couples who used gametes from relatives gave feedback. In general, the donation was seen to equalize genetic parenthood and help legitimize the woman's motherhood. No legislation exists regarding donations by relatives, but the American Society for Reproductive Medicine (ASRM) Ethics Committee in a 2012 statement concluded that intrafamilial gamete donors behave ethically when all participants are fully informed and counseled.

IS SURROGACY ETHICAL?

The American Society for Reproductive Medicine (ASRM) Ethics Committee also permits surrogacy but stipulates that participants should receive additional counseling to ensure they make free informed decisions. Experts know that patients sometimes ignore informed-consent documents, considering them empty rituals that are difficult to decipher. However, at least one study of donors shows that women know exactly what they are doing when they consent. University of California,

San Francisco, researchers applied the Egg Donor Informed Consent Tool to 22 donors and found average scores fell in the mid-90 percent range and did not differ with the woman's age, education, race, or ethnicity.

According to Seton Hall University law student Jill Colban (2016), although gestational surrogacy (no genetic connection between surrogate and baby) is the procedure of choice today in most clinics, both traditional surrogacy and gestational surrogacy pose ethical and moral concerns. First, the payment of services to the surrogate can be equated to baby selling, which is illegal, and then the surrogate's service is diminished since her role is reduced to a commodity ("rent a womb").

Also, sometimes African American or minority women are exploited as surrogates more than Caucasians since ART services can demand a high fee and women in lower socioeconomic situations need money. Thus, the ethical principle of justice or fairness does not apply here. One way to solve this ethical dilemma is to permit only altruistic surrogacy. This not only reduces the risk of economic exploitation but also eliminates racial bias.

Some experts believe women are unable to grasp the huge psychological and emotional attachment risk of carrying a child over a nine-month period, so some experts build in a "wait period." Feminists could argue that equal rights give women autonomy to choose their lifestyle, and telling a prospective surrogate who has already received informed consent to wait dehumanizes her and imposes a new form of paternalism in which she must consult a man before agreeing to bear a child. Women require equal amounts of autonomy and justice if they are to apply ethical decisions.

How Many IVF Cycles Are Ethical?

Miriam Zoll, author of *Cracked Open*, says in the Netflix documentary *Future Babies* that after the age of 37, women lose 90–95 percent of their eggs. How ethical is it then for doctors to hold out hope to older women that they will conceive when they have only a 6–10 percent chance of succeeding in IVF?

Wendy Vitek, a reproductive endocrinologist at the University of Rochester Medical Center in New York State, verifies that the rates for individual cycles generally decline with each successive attempt. For older women aged 40–42, the first cycle of IVF returns a success rate of 12.3 percent; a second cycle falls to 10.1 percent, and by the ninth cycle, there are no live births for this age group. Moreover, how ethical is it for women to undergo more than four or five IVF cycles? In the United States IVF takes enormous financial resources, emotional strength, and perseverance, not to mention stamina. Where is the beneficence in encouraging a woman to keep repeating a procedure with no real benefits and considerable risks?

In 2016, U.K. researcher Dr. Scott Nelson told Creating a Family, a national infertility and adoption education nonprofit, that two-thirds of women younger than 40 will achieve a live birth after five or six treatment cycles but stipulate the cutoff age at 40. Administering IVF to women over age 40 reflects questionable ethics unless the woman is using younger donated eggs.

ETHICS OF U.S. NONREGULATION

As stated in Chapter 5, Jessica Schneider volunteered as a three-time egg donor but died of cancer at age 31. Her doctor said it was possible that the fertility hormones she took caused her cancer. Jessica was victimized by an economic system that puts money ahead of the health of the individual donor. Fertility clinics perform a valuable service but depend on egg suppliers, who are compensated monetarily. For that financial reason, both the clinics and women do not want regulatory limits imposed on them. However, there may be serious physical risks to repeated egg harvesting.

Mildred Cho of Stanford University Center for Biomedical Ethics in California says that more research needs to be done to uncover the risks of egg harvesting. Danielle A. Vera writes in the *Michigan Journal of Gender and Law* that donors are lured into a manipulative situation because doctors have a conflict of interest between good medical service and the huge profits reaped from egg donors. Danielle Vera says this lack of ethics justifies a greater need for government intervention to study the long-term effects of egg harvesting.

The Food and Drug Administration (FDA) has so far kept a hands-off approach on ART by emphasizing the autonomy of the doctor-patient relationship. Some states have various regulations, but none limit the number of eggs or cycles that each supplier is permitted to sell. In Vera's article she states that the process of getting informed consent from egg suppliers is seriously "deficient." In other words, women do not get a full picture of their risks and rewards.

Due to lack of governmental regulation, unethical policies prevail. States do not stipulate how many children may be conceived from one donor, what types of medical information or updates must be supplied by donors, what genetic tests may be performed on embryos, how many fertilized eggs may be placed in a woman, or how old a donor can be. The lack of these regulations can negatively affect patients and families.

Take, for instance, the number of times a donor's sperm or eggs are used to conceive a child. Parents should know that number, says Naomi Cahn, a George Washington University law professor. The concern here is that offspring of a frequent donor could inadvertently meet and fall in love, raising the possibility of "accidental incest." Nonmaleficence in the form of disclosure of the extent of gamete use is necessary to maintain ethical health care.

Also, fraudulent or skewed practices of clinics in reporting success rates can significantly affect parents-to-be. Some clinics may report higher success rates because they transfer more embryos—not because they necessarily have more live births. Clinics also can cancel cycles prior to egg retrieval when there is a low oocyte response to stimulation. Moreover, clinics have monetary and reporting incentives to utilize IVF early in treatment rather than to explore less expensive and potentially effective options like artificial insemination (AI). In doing this, they inflate rates by including patients who would have gotten pregnant without IVF.

Data from the Centers for Disease Control and Prevention (CDC; cited by the Oakland, California, *Tribune*) said 80 percent of U.S. fertility clinics in 2006—the most recent year for which records are available—did not follow embryo implant guidelines set in 1999 by ASRM. ASRM advises implanting no more than two embryos in women younger than 35, but if it means more money or better success rates, ART clinics often disregard ethical self-regulation by rejecting counsel from professional societies.

eSET versus Double Embryo Transplant
Why Parents Still Want Multiple Transfers

As many as 63 clinics in the United States fail to implement single embryo transfers (SET) in younger women. One reason is patients prefer two embryos or twins. Other reasons are the perception of higher live birth rates with the transfer of two or more embryos (double embryo transplant; DET) and the risk of a high dropout rate from failed SET cycles due to financial, emotional, and/or physical reasons. Physicians sometimes consent to multiple transfers to inflate their success rates. Physicians tend to suggest SET only if there is a lack of competition in their geographic area. Also, fertility doctors believe the risk data on multiples are not compelling enough despite the ASRM and Society for Assisted Reproductive Technology (SART) SET guidelines.

Additional incentives to multiple transfer are the high out-of-pocket costs associated with repeated IVF cycles and the limited insurance coverage for most U.S. patients as well as patients' general lack of knowledge about the risks and complications associated with multiple births.

Still, eSET is not without its risks. Few women receive informed consent and counseling that eSET provides a greater risk for multiple births than a traditional pregnancy and that eSET increases the risk of the embryo splitting into multiple identical children—twin rates are around 1–2 percent

Thus, researchers concluded that mandatory SET is not justified and that many countries should reconsider their current embryo transfer policy. For example, Hungary, Switzerland, India, and Italy limit the number of embryos that can be transferred to three; France and Japan generally limit to two embryos while Sweden, Belgium, Turkey, and Quebec require eSET for most transfers. In contrast, other countries such as the United States and United Kingdom do not currently regulate the number of transfers.

Application of Ethics—Autonomy

From an ethical standpoint, which procedure—eSET or DET—is better? Under the ethical umbrella of autonomy, women seemingly have the last word in determining what procedure they want, though physicians have greater autonomy since they choose the best embryo using preimplantation genetic diagnosis (PGD). (And their paternalism has credibility since 600 common recessive autosomal diseases can be tested to ensure embryo health.)

Physicians, however, may overprioritize patient autonomy (to have twins or two embryos) and ignore or undervalue other ethical considerations. For example, in multiple transfers, patients may have to deal with the ethical hot button of abortion (selective reduction). Also, a policy of refusing DET to women because it is not in their best interests would be clearly paternalistic and interfere with people's choice of what they should do with their bodies. It would constitute a severe infringement on a woman's property rights or autonomy.

Application of Ethics—Beneficence

Beneficent aspects include avoiding risks to women's health associated with carrying multiple embryos. These risks include preeclampsia (a condition characterized by high blood pressure, fluid retention, and proteinuria), placental previs (when the placenta partially or wholly blocks the neck of the uterus), preterm premature rupture of the membranes, cesarean delivery, gestational diabetes, placental abruption (separation of the placenta from the wall of the uterus), and postpartum hemorrhage. Studies show that eSET in women under 37 resulted in increased live births compared with multiple transfers. Even in women aged 37–40, the live birth rate in eSET group was similar to that in the multiple transfer group (DET). And for older women (40+) eSET reduces multiple birth rates but has no other benefit.

Another benefit is DET results in the live birth of extra individuals (approximately 5 extra children for every 10 live-born children from SET). Thus, a reanalysis of the financial costs favors DET, costing approximately $3,790 less per live birth compared with eSET.

Fertility specialist Kelton Tremellen and his colleagues posed the question whether mandating eSET is ethically justifiable in young women. Several areas—for instance, Sweden, Belgium, Turkey, and Quebec—have legally mandated eSET for young women due to complications

(*Reproductive BioMedicine and Society Online*, 2016). These areas mandated SET based on the principle of beneficence, which requires that doctors apply the "do no harm" injunction. On the other hand, two distinct advantages or benefits emerge from DET: twinning from a parental perspective has gained favor due to one pregnancy and one period of child-rearing, which is less disruptive to a woman's career and earning potential than two pregnancies and two periods of maternity leave. As for psychosocial effects, although an analysis from the children's perspective is lacking, it is fair to say that mothers with twins pay less attention and give less nurturance to each individual child than mothers with singletons. So multiple children may be on the losing end.

Application of Ethics—Justice

Another ethical principle is distributive justice, which states that SET should be mandated for all young women because of the increased costs of caring for mothers and babies from complications related to twin delivery. Some ethicists suggest that any increased risk to a child is ethically unacceptable (since both doctors and parents have a moral obligation to act in the child's best interests). However, doctors and parents sometimes behave in a potentially unfair way. For example, parents can decline immunization of their children, and mothers who take drugs or drink excessive amounts of alcohol during pregnancy are not incarcerated.

Application of Ethics—Nonmaleficence

Ethics dictate that if parental choices do not rise to the level of abuse, parents can risk DET. However, significant costs fall on hospitals, the state, and society from the decision to undergo DET versus SET. For example, one estimate based on the number of IVF twins in the United States puts the total annual additional cost at almost $1 billion. Do the expenses for all those extra births balance society's benefits of parenting twins?

Multiple births also place heavy psychosocial effects on the family, with members exhibiting such symptoms as depression, anxiety, relationship stress, and financial stress. In a paper in *Theories of Medical Bioethics* (Wilkinson et al., April 2015) researchers assessed three arguments in favor of mandatory SET: risks to the mother, risks to resultant children, and costs to society. The growing consensus to implant one rather than two embryos results from the fact that complications requiring neonatal care are more common with DETs. Some children get hurt. Is the maleficence of DET strong enough to justify overriding the woman's autonomy?

Another question that must pass ethical muster is whether the transfer of a poor-quality embryo together with a good-quality embryo affects the IVF outcome, as posited in the *Journal of Ovarian Research*

(Wintner et al., 2017). The researchers found that a poor-quality embryo in a total of 603 women does not negatively affect a good-quality embryo when transferred together in a DET. These results contradicted another study that found that transferring an impaired quality embryo along with a good-quality embryo—rather than transferring the good-quality embryo alone—significantly lowered both the pregnancy rates and the implantation rates.

ETHICS FOR SINGLES, HIV PATIENTS, AND LGBTQ (Q STANDS FOR "QUEER") PATIENTS

ASRM states that unmarried or LGBT patients should not be denied fertility services, but menopausal women—not premature menopausal cases—should be discouraged. As for HIV-positive patients, about 3 percent of U.S. clinical practices registered with SART provide services to them. The percentage is so low because some programs and clinics are concerned about risks of transmission to clinic personnel and to other eggs, sperm, and embryos at the clinic. Furthermore, clinic overhead and insurance rates factor into the decision due to the need to provide separate laboratory space and equipment to lower the risk of cross contamination.

The European Society for Human Reproduction and Embryology (ESHRE) Task Force on Ethics and Law stresses that denying access to any of the above groups (defined as "non-standard" situations and relationships) cannot be reconciled with a human rights perspective. It implies discrimination. Furthermore, practitioners who, because of conscientious objection, refuse to assist in ART should refer these patients to other professionals willing to assist. For instance, fertility preservation should be offered to transsexual people considering sex reassignment with counseling by a psychologist with relevant experience.

If doctors treat nonstandard applicants, they have the moral responsibility to invest in follow-up studies for data collection. If there are concerns about the implications of ART on the well-being of anyone involved, including the future child, a surrogate mother, or the applicants themselves, these concerns must be considered in the light of current scientific evidence. When doing so, it is important to avoid the use of double standards such as lesbian and gay parents are competent to raise children, but transgenders are not.

ETHICS OF POSTHUMOUS HARVESTING

Professional societies such as ESHRE and ASRM agree that posthumous sperm conception should only occur in the presence of explicit written consent from the deceased man. However, this can be impractical as many deaths of reproductive-age men are sudden and unexpected, precluding explicit consent. Therefore, medical organizations recognize a standard of presumed consent for posthumous conception with provisions for men to opt out and safeguards to protect the welfare of the prospective mother and her child. The ethical bottom line is physicians should support the rights and welfare of the living (widow and prospective child), not the dead.

In a 2011 study by the National Agricultural Library, Gary S. Nakhuda and his colleagues examined couples' degrees of agreement on postmortem sperm retrieval. Approximately 78 percent of the 106 participating couples stated they would permit PAR (posthumous assisted reproduction). Most of the couples correctly predicted their mates' attitudes. Nakhuda concluded that while most ART individuals would agree to PAR, a portion would not consent.

Angela Lawson writes in the *European Journal of Contraception and Reproductive Health Care* (2016) that although PAR can be viewed unfavorably by some people, many individuals whose partners die of cancer or another illness prior to the completion of family building may desire PAR. PAR is technically feasible for males and females (both premortem and postmortem), and these procedures have been completed on numerous occasions and are always guided by the ethical concepts of autonomy, beneficence, and justice for the living, the deceased, and the soon-to-be conceived. Furthermore, psychological risks to PAR can affect all parties. As such, beneficence dictates early psychological counseling of patients and surviving family members.

ETHICS OF HUMAN CLONING

Eight in 10 American adults (81 percent) say cloning a human being is not morally acceptable, according to a May 2016 Gallup poll and Pew Research. Since 2001, overwhelming opposition to human cloning has existed. Just 13 percent of adults in 2016 said cloning is morally acceptable. About 46 countries have formally banned human cloning, but the United States has no laws referring to it.

Henry Greely (*The End of Sex*) says human cloning would appeal only to a minority. Also, it is unclear whether it would ever become safe enough. About 20 species of mammals have been cloned, and for some creatures such as mice, it has become routine, but physicians and scientists from the American Medical Association (AMA) and American Association for the Advancement of Science (AAAS) have issued formal public statements on its potential for danger and ethical irresponsibility.

As with many hotly debated ethical issues, scientists, researchers, and the public often differ. According to Sophia M. Kolehmainen, a lawyer with the Cambridge, Massachusetts-based Council for Responsible Genetics, cloning improves the production of genetically engineered animals, but human cloning would be a mistake. For one thing, a period of human experimentation would yield partially successful humans just as the cloned sheep Dolly originally produced 276 failed lambs. The loss of animals may be ethically acceptable, but human failures would not be.

Second, cloning encourages the commodification of humans, turning procreation into manufacturing. Third, cloning would disrespect human diversity in ethnicity and ability, and fourth, it would invite permanent changes to the gene pool, a dangerous event that might open the door to eugenics. Animal cloning might improve inherited characteristics, but human eugenics would not necessarily improve character traits. According to genetics experts, cloning is not a cure for infertility; it is a replication of something that already exists.

Author Joshua May writes in *Reproductive Ethics* (2015) that adults are repulsed, curious, and anxious about human cloning, but whatever their reaction, they also feel it is immoral, unethical, and should be illegal. Lee Silver, professor of genetics at Princeton University, sees the ethical problem as creating a gap between parental haves and parental have-nots. The haves will pay for gene advantages for their children like longevity and decreased risks of cancer, stroke, and dementia; the have-nots will be unable to afford it. Also, parents think they will be able to increase the behavioral and cognitive aspects of their children and possibly their talents, but cloning only increases possibilities. How then will parents feel when their children do not express the special genes that they received? Also, Greely says clones would not be as similar as identical twins despite their almost identical DNA. They would not have developed inside the same uterus or been raised in the same physical and cultural environment.

CONCLUSION

The fact that few regulations govern ART permits the rules of conduct to be looser than in other areas in which parents, physicians, and children interact, but they still must pass muster with the four pillars of ethics, such as autonomy and beneficence. Doctors over the past 25 years have implanted multiple embryos in women, authorized a high number of fertility trials, and, in the name of justice, allowed several nontraditional groups to participate (such as single women/men, gays, lesbians, and transgenders). Physicians nowadays are still debating the ethics of growing trends toward donated eggs and surrogacy by relatives and eSET rather than multiple transfers. Thanks to PGD, eSET is a safer option.

Commercialized surrogacy was allowed for a time and is still permitted in many areas of the United States and other countries, but gestational surrogacy is now more the ethical rule as is altruistic surrogacy. Also, posthumous collection of gametes has become ethically acceptable. The next chapter deals again with ethics, but these moral decisions relate to the children of ART procedures.

CHAPTER 9

Is ART Compatible with Children's Rights?

This chapter explains the ethics governing children's rights in Assisted Reproductive Technology (ART). How can parents and physicians maintain the health of a fetus or fetuses in a multipregnancy? How can selective reduction of embryos be ethical? What principles or value systems prioritize children and their rights as embryos, fetuses, and live births? Do children have a right to not live? Do children have the right to hold physicians and parents responsible for genetic diseases that are not scanned for? What about the ethics of gene therapy such as mitochondrial gene therapy (MGT), clustered regularly interspace short palindromic repeats (CRISPR), and next-generation sequencing NGS?

PARENTAL AGE

Children have a right to be born safely to a mother healthy enough to care for them until they reach the age of majority, but older mothers—women over 40—are at higher risk for many medical problems. For instance, they are twice as likely to suffer a stillbirth or miscarriage. Also, older mothers are between three and six times more likely to die in the six weeks following the birth of the baby due to complications such as bleeding and clots.

More than half of women over age 40 will require cesarean section, a risky procedure for both mother and child. Finally, babies born from older mothers are 1.5–2 times more likely to be born premature and with a low birth weight. This carries an immediate risk of lung problems for the babies and later, the risks of obesity and diabetes as adults.

Infants of older mothers are at risk too if their mother consents to implanting several embryos. The babies can be born early (preterm) and have a host of serious problems including low birth weight, respiratory distress syndrome, sepsis, jaundice, developmental delays, neural tube defects, heart malformations, bronchopulmonary dysplasia, spontaneous abortion, and cerebral palsy.

Prospective fathers' ages also can influence their children's right to health. When Harvard researchers looked at nearly 19,000 IVF cycles among 7,753 couples between 2000 and 2014, they found that the likelihood of a live birth declined with the increasing age of the male partner. Also, a Swedish study in 2014 indicated that fathers older than 45 are more likely to have children with schizophrenia, autism, and other psychiatric disorders. Late-age fathers triggered achondroplasia or dwarfism in one of 2,000 births.

Besides these physical results, older parents inevitably force their young children and teen-aged sons and daughters to prematurely care for aging parents with disabilities such as heart disease, diabetes, and dementia. Is it morally right for a young child to have to deal with this burden?

DISABILITY RIGHTS

In 2016 an Australian couple with Down syndrome sought ART to start a family. Their parents did not approve, but disability advocates argued that intellectually impaired people should have the same rights as others in the community, and their right to health does not preclude marriage and reproduction.

It follows then that if children have the right to health, the flip side to this is their right to disability. Ethicists argue that this right to disability is an essential component of individual autonomy and the right to an open future in which a child's opportunities in life are not limited. Some deaf parents would prefer children with that same disability since they regard it as using their autonomy to create a better, easier parenting relationship. Bioethicists often side with disability activists on this point. They agree that technological advances (such as gene editing) may reflect the view of disability as an abnormality instead of a natural feature of human diversity. In citing the Americans with Disabilities Act (ADA), bioethicists agree that disabled persons are not inferior and should not suffer discrimination, no matter the severity of the disability.

For example, American poet Sheila Black unknowingly passed on her disability—X-linked hypophosphatemia or a form of dwarfism—to two of her three children. The genetic counselor had told Black not to worry about transmitting her condition, but the counselor's calculations were incorrect, and gene mapping had not progressed to a point of accuracy yet. Still, Black says she never regretted having children with a disability despite knowing they suffer both physical and psychic pain. Her attitude is calm acceptance of their uniqueness, and the children themselves speak of their disability in positive ways—that it taught them empathy and that fitting in with the group is not the only path to happiness. In this case, justice and beneficence prevailed since the mother and children feel contented and on a level playing field with others.

One reason disabled women like Black allow a disabled child to be born is they do not always receive up-to-date reproductive healthcare information due to poor access to mobility devices, public transportation, or computers. Many in the medical professions still deem disabled persons unsuitable for reproduction because doctors and other experts say they are unable to care for their children adequately. The result is disabled women often receive less information. The ethical dispute over disability has not been resolved yet. While mainstream society rejects disability in terms of the four basic principles of healthcare ethics, disability activists often embrace the ethical uniqueness of their disability and their children's.

EMBRYO/CHILD TREATMENT

Has PGD negatively affected growing children? When researchers studied six-year-old PGD-screened children at the Centre for Medical Genetics in Brussels, they found they did not suffer from problem behaviors and their psychosocial development compared favorably with the control group (Winter et al., *Human Reproduction*, May 2015). Beneficence prevailed.

In contrast, when compared with singletons, children produced from multiple births are associated with an increased risk of poor parenting and a reported compromise in quality of life. An increased risk of child abuse arises in families raising multiples, particularly when one or more of the children have special needs. Multiple births can trigger maleficent warnings like "Do no harm."

The Octomom

What better way to illustrate the ethics (or lack thereof) of multifetal ART than to reexamine the "octomom" case. In the *Journal of Clinical Research & Bioethics* (2011) Manninen discusses the moral dimensions of Californian Nadya Suleman's actions, starting with her procreative liberty or right to biologically produce children. This right, however, needed to be exercised in a morally valid way. In applying and weighing the four main ethical principles related to her behavior, Suleman's actions favor the unethical. Suleman, her physician, insurance companies, and even the media shared responsibility for shortchanging the children. This social connection model, according to political theorist and feminist Iris Marion Young, dictates that those who participate in or benefit from some unjust or harmful outcome are responsible for taking steps to rectify the wrong and ensure it will not reoccur.

Suleman applied her moral duty of self-improvement to bear and raise children, but by implanting six embryos, this action conflicted with the duty of parental responsibility. She put her own desires for a large family before the welfare of her existing and newly born children. She disregarded health risks (disabilities in infants) as well as economics. In addition, Suleman ignored the medical dangers of a multiple birth; the negative impact that eight additional children would have on an already large family; and her lack of financial, emotional, and mental resources. In short, she failed to act in a responsible, judicious, and virtuous manner for the sake of her children.

Suleman's doctor also failed in his ethical challenges but defended his actions by citing his patient's procreative and ownership rights. However, he indulged his patient's desire to implant too many embryos, allowing his patient's decision (autonomy) to prevail instead of opting for medical benefi- cence or medical paternalism. The physician had a duty to avoid harming the children, and in this case, it should have trumped Suleman's reproductive autonomy. His role as a fertility doctor and his ethic of care were to act responsibly when implanting the embryos. He violated that. Second, he allowed even greater health risks by initiating fresh cycles instead of using frozen embryos. (Data presented at the 2013 American Society for Repro- ductive Medicine (ASRM) annual meeting found that women of advanced maternal age had a significantly higher live birth rate using frozen embryos compared to fresh embryos—74.5 percent versus 53.7 percent.)

The fertility physicians comprise one group in the social connection model. Marion Young says due to the trust that patients put in doctors, fer- tility physicians have a responsibility to limit the uses of ARTs that lead to multiple births. Also, insurance companies share in this responsibility because their policies play a vital role in patients' decisions concerning treatment. Many studies confirmed that when insurance covers all fertility treatments, patients are relieved of the financial pressures and are less likely to implant three or more embryos. Also, patients without insurance use intrauterine insemination (IUI) twice as frequently as IVF because it is cheaper, but this usage limits the control on the number of implanted embryos. One study found that in states that do not mandate medical cov- erage of fertility treatments, they have the highest number of embryos transferred per IVF cycle and a higher percentage of live multiple births than states that require partial or complete coverage.

Even the media share in an ethical responsibility to the children. Reporters often depict an unrealistic picture of multiple births since they tend to skip over sad scenarios of premature infants dying of painful dis- eases or suffering from long-term disabilities. Instead they present an idealized view of healthy "miracle" children. Also, they neglect to inform the public of the high hospital bills and traumatic pediatric treatments.

ADOPTED OR ABANDONED EMBRYOS

The Ethics Committee of the ASRM issues reports on several ART- related issues. For example, the committee believes the term "embryo adoption" is deceptive because it points to the embryo as a fully entitled legal being when it should not be viewed as such. The committee also counseled against telling offspring of their donor conception since it may subject the child to social and psychological turmoil.

Another ethical opinion relates to the disposition of abandoned embryos. The committee supports disclosure of the preimplantation genetic diagnosis (PGD) screening of embryos, which usually results in extra embryos. According to the Ethics Committee, women of advanced reproductive age should not receive adopted embryos since their risk level opens the door to pregnancy loss and other obstetric complications as well as potential harm to children.

FORCED GENE ANALYSIS

PGD, even when used only to screen out and eliminate the sick or "deficient," may change parents' attitudes toward their children, increasing both the desire to control and the tacit expectation of certain qualities. This attitude might intensify as PGD becomes more sophisticated and Health Maintenance Organizations (HMOs) or health plans that cover IVF require PGD to prevent certain costly diseases.

Questionable PGD

Ethics are even harder to determine when transferring embryos with indeterminate PGD results. In a 2016 paper in *Fertility Research and Ethic Practice* the authors discuss how physicians need to create action plans because PGD results show a 7.5 percent rate of inconclusive results. For instance, a case study involving a 39-year-old *BRCA-1* (cancer) carrier who needed IVF to eliminate his male factor infertility opted for PGD to select against *BRCA-1* gene carrier embryos (hereditary breast and ovarian cancer). However, several embryos were returned with inconclusive results, and the couple proceeded with the transfer of these embryos.

The above case was presented before the ART Ethics Committee, which debated the physician's duty to protect patient autonomy, to act in the best interests of the future child and to benefit society. The transfer of known-carrier embryos (cancer causing) was felt to be unethical for certain disease states depending on the severity of illness and the timing of disease onset. However, no overarching guidelines or consensus regarding embryos with indeterminate carrier status exist. The ESHRE Task Force opines that physicians should only refuse to assist patients in their reproductive efforts if the quality of life of the child is so low that it would have been better off not to have been born.

Not everyone, however, concludes that PGD has the moral foundation for informed consent. One criticism is that PGD is dehumanizing and transforms birth into a commodity since the entire process revolves around the transfer of procreation from the home to the laboratory. Another criticism is that not everyone can afford the add-on IVF test, thus negating the ethical principle of justice or rendering to others what should be due.

ETHICS OF NEWER TECHNIQUES

Mitochondrial DNA

Mitochondrial disease can be transmitted through the mitochondrial DNA in 37 genes in women. Both sexes of children can inherit it, but only women are at risk of transmitting it. According to Rebecca Dimond of the Cardiff School of Social Sciences, United Kingdom, about 1 in 400 people carry a mitochondrial mutation that produces a disease. Mitochondrial disease is extremely variable, and patients can be mildly, severely, or fatally affected. Symptoms include diabetes, epilepsy, digestive disorders, fatigue, cardiomyopathy, deafness, restricted sight, and difficulties with mobility and balance.

The biggest ethical problem with mitochondrial replacement therapy (MRT) is the creation of three-parent babies, a result that complicates legal parentage rights. The courts have thus far relied on "intent" to award parentage rights, but with MRT, relying on intent could reasonably result in the recognition of three legal parents since all three contributors "intended" to have the child. However, Amy Leiser in *The Georgetown Law Journal* (2016) concludes that the intent test is still the best way to resolve disputes because it can be applied without regard to gender or amount of DNA contributed. This avoids discrimination and invokes the principle of justice. The intent test is also flexible and adapts to changing circumstances such as increased uses of MRT. Best of all it ends the problem of legal parentage, which could prevent the use of MRT for women who desperately need it to have healthy children.

Bonnie Rochman in *The Gene Machine* (Scientific American, 2017) explains that MRT involves replacing defective mitochondria in the IVF-produced embryo with healthy genetic material. She cites a successful 2016 case in which a New York City physician performed MRT to prevent a woman from transferring the neurological disease Leigh syndrome to her baby. Despite the positive result, in 2016, as mentioned previously, the Food and Drug Administration (FDA) amended its recommendation of MRT for special cases and said that until proven safe, only male embryos should receive the transferred mitochondria since only women pass along mitochondrial DNA.

Mitochondrial gene replacement also favors the help/harm ratio. Since thousands of mothers could potentially harm their offspring by transmitting mitochondrial diseases, transmission prevention is the only current hope. In an article about MRT and CRISPR by Sarah Fogleman et al.

(*American Journal of Stem Cells*, 2016) the authors look at the risk benefit ratio for MRT donors. Risks to those donating include daily hormonal injections and added stress from the relatively invasive procedure. The process of hormone injections also raises the risk of ovarian hypersti-mulation syndrome. Another ethical obstacle is the lack of long-term research into how MRT will affect the offspring and subsequent genera-tions. A 2017 study in *Nature* suggested that about 15 percent of cases could fail and allow fatal defects to return or even increase a child's sus-ceptibility to new ailments. One of the biggest ethical concerns for MRT is the argument that doctors are playing God by changing the DNA.

In the United Kingdom, the ethical determination differs from that of the United States. The U.K. Department of Health does not accept that the MRT child will have three parents because the genes contributing to personal characteristics and traits come solely from the nuclear DNA, which only comes from the proposed child's mother and father. The donated mitochondrial DNA does not affect those characteristics. Thus, according to the United Kingdom's ethical interpretation, the rela-tionship between child and donor eliminates any legal obligation on the donor's part because there is no significant genetic relationship between the child and donor. The U.K. Health Department compares MRT to a tis-sue/organ donation.

CRISPR/Cas9

Another novel gene-editing technique called CRISPR/Cas9 uses the principles of bacterial immune function to target and remove specific sequences of mutated DNA. It can help with a donor embryo (using three-parent IVF) by transplanting the patient's nuclear DNA to the blastocyst.

The gene-editing technology known as CRISPR is making ethicists more nervous than MRT. CRISPR allows scientists to edit the genome by removing, replacing, or adding to parts of the DNA sequence. Many people worry that this is the entryway to the horrors of eugenics that scien-tists have been debating and debasing for years. For one thing designer babies using CRISPR would mean parents could engineer disabilities into their child's genome. On the plus side, this might permanently destigma-tize disabilities—something disability activists have wanted for years.

If CRISPR is not regulated, people could easily argue that parents and offspring have as much a right to disability as a right to health. As stated earlier the right to disability, such as deafness or dwarfism, is a direct descendant of the ADA. Although most parents would rather give birth to a hearing child or one of normal height, there are parents who feel they are more capable to raise a child "like them."

In contrast, CRISPR could also be used to secure a right to health and an "open future" for children. For example, a prospective child has a right to life above a predetermined reasonable threshold, and parents owe children a right to autonomy—to possess the right not to suffer certain disabilities that fall below a reasonable threshold of harm. Most potential parents would probably use CRISPR to eradicate genetic disease, but ethics might be cast aside. Could potential parents decide not to use CRISPR and permit genetic diseases to happen naturally? Could potential parents be permitted to use it to impose disability on their prospective children? Are all disabilities equal in the eyes of society, or could we redesign our population's range of disability? A multitude of ethical questions might result from the continued lack of regulation.

So far CRISPR has revolutionized the modification of the genomes of bacteria, plants, and animals. First described in 1993 in a bacterium from a salt marsh, by 2014 it was used for gene editing in a wide range of organisms from yeasts to monkeys. It became a worldwide venture involving scientists in nine different countries.

In 2015 Chinese scientists made a major step forward. With CRISPR, which makes it cheaper and easier to alter the DNA inside cells, prospective parents could choose which DNA variations their children would have. Then a technique could be used to remove or inactivate defective genes, correct mutations, or even replace genes. Not only could parents avoid an undesirable genetic disease or trait, but they also could use genomic engineering to add other enhancements that may emerge in the next 20–40 years.

Currently genome editing is used in a small number of exceptional life-threatening cases to replace defective genes with new healthy ones and significantly reduce the number of patients suffering from cardiac problems, diabetes, and many genetically transmitted diseases such as cystic fibrosis, sickle cell anemia, and some cancers. According to *Medical Discovery News*, genome editing is more a gentle tweak in the right direction; CRISPR is faster, cheaper, and more accurate, acting as a pair of "molecular scissors" so that bits or single nucleotide polymorphisms (SNP) chips of DNA can be added or removed. (In late 2007 SNP chips became more common in research and were used by a firm called 23andMe to offer ancestry information.)

While many people criticize and are shocked at the use of PGD, the gene-editing technique CRISPR is closer to the ambivalent desire for designer babies. CRISPR uses the protein Cas9 to find an individual defective DNA sequence and repair the mistake. Thus, this biological editing skill has the potential to fix many genetic diseases, such as liver disease.

In 2016 Chinese researchers tried to use CRISPR to make nonviable embryos resistant to HIV, but too many difficulties precluded success. China has continued to progress, according to clinicaltrials.gov. In 2017 China headed 9 trials out of the 10 listed. Three of the experimental groups confirmed to *Science* that the Chinese are infusing cancer patients with their own immune cells modified using CRISPR.

CRISPR is a work in progress. Questions about the procedure abound. Even the invention of this technique is confusing. Usually traced to 2012 and Jennifer Doudna at University of California Berkeley and Emmanuelle Charpentier, controversy over the true inventors has produced a patent fight. Still, CRISPR has been widely and enthusiastically adopted by laboratories around the world. Also, another technique called gene silencing may eventually be useful in turning off dangerous genes that cause conditions in people. A German study hopes to be able to use gene silencing to stop Huntington's disease, a neurodegenerative disease.

Nathaniel Comfort, author of *The Science of Human Perfection* (Yale University Press, 2012), says the technology of CRISPR will tinker with embryos, but he believes that it probably will not work the way people think it will. A parent may want to increase a child's IQ, but who knows what else that gene does. Katrine Bosley, CEO of gene-editing company Editas Medicine, says the near future will probably focus on more meaningful outcomes. For example, scientists may want to cure a disease, but slowing or stopping its progress might be the kind of realistic advances they should look forward to.

Editas is working only on somatic cell disease, which is confined to cells other than egg or sperm. Changes to somatic cells are not passed on to future generations as are changes to germ cells (egg or sperm), so this reduces some of the ethical challenges that have stirred objections about the slippery slope of eugenics.

In CRISPR the embryos would have to be tested, and the more cells that are singled out, the greater possibility of incomplete editing and mosaicism. This method would use a lot of embryos, and the unsuccessful editing of otherwise healthy embryos and the destruction of those improperly edited would be a moral problem for many people and not just pro-lifers. CRISPR technology could even be used for evil purposes such as breeding killer mosquitoes or spreading viruses that destroy agriculture.

The world of ART is changing at a rapid pace, and prominent geneticist George Church has already said that CRISPR is en route to becoming "old stuff." Rather than edit genomes, Church poses the challenge of constructing artificial ones. A group called "Human Genome Project-Write" intends to make human DNA from chemicals, which theoretically would allow scientists to manufacture a human genome immune to viruses and even synthesize a human being without biological parents.

Next-Generation Sequencing

Next-generation sequencing (NGS) is PGD improved, so it reveals an even more detailed examination of chromosomes. More cost effective than the current PGD, high-resolution NGS reveals a wider range of mosaic embryos—those that contain a mixture of normal and abnormal cells. High-resolution NGS has the potential to provide the whole genome sequence of an embryo, enabling detection of chromosome count as well as defects.

NGS is already available, at least in special cases. The first baby using hr-NGS was born in 2013. Connor Levy was part of an international study at Oxford University in England. His parents had already tried IUI three times without success. After they signed up for IVF at a Pennsylvania clinic, the couple was offered NGS, which was developed to read whole genomes quickly and cheaply. The mother produced 13 embryos, but Oxford specialists discovered that only 3 had the right number of chromosomes. Her doctor implanted one embryo, and nine months later Connor was born. Pennsylvania fertility physician Michael Glassner believes NGS is a revolutionary procedure that will increase pregnancy rates by 50 percent across the board and reduce miscarriages by a similar margin. This state-of-the-art technology is coming soon to your neighborhood fertility clinic provided the United States retains its nonregulatory policies.

CONCLUSION

Ethics governing children's rights help define the risk-benefit of different ART procedures such as selective reduction, multiple high-order pregnancies, and parental age. All these factors have positive and negative ramifications for children depending on the ethical standards applied, such as the help-harm ratio, beneficence, distributive justice, and autonomy.

Ethics will get more complicated as PGD starts to address characteristics such as behavior, temperament, and personality, and scientists are able to tweak skin cells into gametes. Heterosexual and homosexual relationships will profit from this as surrogacy rates decrease. Also, if insurance mandates spread to other states, DET will drop out of ART and eSETs will become the gold standard. MRT and NGS changes should improve ART for children and parents, making it safer and more specific.

In Chapter 10, savior siblings are discussed as one of the more controversial products of IVF along with the related psychosocial factors that affect donors as well as recipients. Fertility option will continue to multiply if science has anything to say about it, but what will ethicists make of artificial ovaries and wombs, artificial gametes, and the AUGMENT treatment?

The Ethics of "Savior Siblings"

According to a 2004 survey of more than 6,000 Americans by the Genetics and Public Policy Center at John Hopkins University, twice as many Americans approved of using preimplantation genetic diagnosis (PGD) to select an embryo that could benefit an ailing sibling. Most participants believed there was a moral obligation to use genetic testing if the purpose was to prevent the suffering of a child. This survey validated the right to life of the so-called savior sibling, a baby conceived so that his or her stem cells might save an older sibling from dying of a deadly disease.

This final chapter brings together the role of the savior sibling and the ethics of that position. Thanks to IVF and PGD using blastocysts, parents are now able to choose the best embryo to implant to avoid the genetic disease that an older sibling might have. "Easy PGD" is discussed later in the chapter. Henry T. Greeley, author and Stanford expert in law and biology, coined the name of this gene editing technique, which in concert with stem cell production of gametes could one day possibly eliminate the need for IVF.

MORAL OBLIGATION

Australian researcher Kimberly Strong speaks of the "moral valorization" of savior siblings. Strong says parents have an intuitive grasp of the moral obligation to care for sick children, and what better way than by savior siblings donating stem cells in their umbilical cords to older, sick siblings. When it comes to the ethics of savior siblings, parents take a naturalistic approach. Potential loss, fear, and commodification of another child line up on one side; on the other are relational autonomy, beneficence, and morality.

Morality is what trumps any qualms about creating embryos, most of which will be discarded in the attempt to find the right embryo. Take, for instance, the genetic disease beta-thalassemia. A child with this disease requires lifelong monthly blood transfusions to maintain satisfactory levels of hemoglobin and iron chelation therapy to combat the tendency to iron overload. That is a health burden no parent wants to place on their child.

Enter the savior sibling. In Clamart, France, near Paris, a Turkish family with a thalassemia-affected child screened a dozen embryos in 2011 until they found one that did not carry the gene for thalassemia and was human leukocyte antigen (HLA) compatible. The outcome? The IVF-conceived child was born healthy, and doctors are confident that the stem cells from his discarded umbilical cord will cure his older sister.

U.S. SAVIOR SIBLING SAVES THE DAY

The first savior sibling in the United States was Adam Nash, who was born on August 29, 2000. His six-year-old sister, Molly, suffered from Fanconi anemia, a genetic disorder leading to failing bone marrow production and the eventual destruction of a child's immune system. After Molly's mother underwent four rounds of IVF and PGD, doctors found that one of her embryos provided a perfectly healthy tissue match for Molly. (Siblings have a one in four chances of matching each other based on inheritance of the same HLA genes from their parents.)

When Adam was born, a team of doctors at the University of Minnesota Medical School immediately gathered Adam's placenta and all the cord blood. Molly started chemotherapy to destroy her own bone marrow and a month later received a transfusion of Adam's umbilical cord blood cells. The transplant did not cure her of her condition, but it eliminated her risk for leukemia. She is still likely to suffer Fanconi anemia's other complications, particularly cancers of the mouth and neck, which is why she visits the doctor 35–40 times a year to screen for solid tumor cancers.

Another savior sibling—this one fictitious—appeared in Jodi Picoult's novel *My Sister's Keeper* (Washington Square Press, 2004). This book's premise illustrates how complex the issues surrounding a savior sibling can be. The story depicts how a medical and psychological bond can tether one child to another, exhorting one sibling to donate an organ. Conceived as a marrow donor for her gravely ill sister, Anna Fitzgerald undergoes countless surgeries and medical procedures. Though the older daughter's life has no doubt been prolonged, the decision of Anna's parents has stressed the entire family. When Anna brings the medical situation to a crisis point by suing her parents for emancipation to avoid undergoing a kidney transplant for her sister, the legal battle sets off a court case that threatens to destroy the family for good. Readers realize that donors also face risks.

RISKS AND BENEFITS: DONORS

As portrayed in the Picoult book, child donors conceived as savior siblings may feel psychological pressure from their parents to donate organs and tissue throughout their lives. For example, if the initial umbilical cord blood transplant is not successful, the donors may be asked to donate bone marrow or even a kidney or liver. A study in the *Journal of Pediatric Psychology* (MacLeod et al., 2003) found that child donors who underwent unsuccessful tissue transplants were less likely to benefit psychologically from the experience and more likely to suffer negative effects such as anger, guilt, and blame. This negativity increases when child donors feel neglected by doctors or family members after the transplant.

Many of the child donors in the unsuccessful transplant group state that it was difficult not to feel responsible for their sibling's death, and the development of negative feelings was harder for siblings who lacked adequate emotional support following the death or when the death was directly related to complications resulting from the transplant. Some of the feelings did not develop right away but grew over time. Thus, even child donors who do not immediately show signs of postsurgical depression, anger, guilt, or blame may still suffer years after an unsuccessful transplant. Child donors may experience a loss of sense of self and purpose in life if their sibling dies.

This same study found that children who donated stem cells experienced fear prior to undergoing the medical procedure. Other related studies found that donors may come to resent their sick siblings because of the significant amount of attention they receive from their parents. These feelings of resentment may lead to depression.

Although forcing a newborn baby to donate cord blood does not subject the infant to physical pain (removing the cord and discarding it is standard procedure immediately after birth), a donor child may be asked numerous times to donate tissue and possibly even organs. That can lead to substantial pain, discomfort, and risk. For example, bone marrow donation involves donor risks—to general anesthesia, infection, and blood transfusions. Donating a kidney includes a possible negative reaction to anesthesia, unexpected blood loss, infection, and the possible loss of function in the donor's remaining kidney; and donating a liver can trigger bleeding, infection, bile leakage, adverse reactions to general anesthesia, lung collapse, stomach irritation, scarring on the abdomen, liver failure, and death.

In Jeffrey P. Kahn's *Dying to Donate?* (CNN, January 2002) he describes the dilemma: although the medical benefit to the recipient is great, the donor has the major risk. The question, therefore, is whether the benefit to the donor of seeing a loved one's life saved or health improved, along with the benefit of doing a remarkably good deed, is sufficient to balance the risk the donor is asked to undergo.

Donor IVF children have more emotional issues than naturally conceived children, according to a Cambridge University study of 198 families over seven years (Golombok et al., *Human Reproduction*, 2006). In the first stage of the study parents were found to be hypersensitive to their child's needs. They leaned toward overinvolvement but felt their children were emotionally average. In the second stage of a blind study, teachers were asked to describe the emotional states of the children. Teachers found that the donor IVF children expressed more emotional problems due to greater anxiety from parental oversensitivity.

RISKS AND BENEFITS: RECIPIENTS

Only a small amount of psychological research has been carried out to determine the effects on the ill sibling, but a case could be made for "gift giving." The recipient of a gift often feels obligated to reciprocate, but an ailing child will, of course, not have the opportunity to reciprocate. This may cause the recipient to perpetually feel as if he or she owes the donor something important. This can lead to a decrease in the recipient child's self-esteem and have profound consequences for the sibling relationship.

Drs. Herbert Brown and Martin Kelly conducted one of the few studies assessing the psychological stress that sick siblings experience (*Psychosomatic Medicine*, November/December 1976) before, during, and after a transplant. Their research demonstrates the stages of stress, including reading an explicit consent form and not feeling fully informed; becoming aware of the possibility of death; experiencing the negative physical side effects of the immunosuppressive drugs; feeling emotionally alone due to the need for physical isolation; dreaming about and fearing the procedure as well as extreme anxiety while waiting in isolation to hear whether the transplant has taken; feeling angry, depressed, and at fault if the marrow fails; combining fear and joy at leaving the hospital; and persistently feeling indebted as well as entitled as a survivor.

INFORMED CONSENT

Risks related to the creation of a savior sibling should be articulated clearly in informed consent documents. Informed consent must be secured from patients for all medical procedures—from removal of a basal skin tumor to a heart transplant. If women and men lack adequate information about Assisted Reproductive Technology (ART) risks and benefits, they cannot give genuine written consent. Clinical psychologist Andrea Mechanick Braverman, who screens egg donors in Philadelphia, says she worries that some women underestimate the invasiveness of ART procedures and long-term emotional ramifications.

Currently, there is no fertility registry that reports risks and problems of IVF or savior children, so women must depend on the forthrightness of fertility doctors and clinics. Reputable clinics supply key risk information as does the 16-page pamphlet from Northwestern University Medicine's Fertility and Reproductive Medicine Clinic. Some clinics hesitate to clarify ART's negative side effects, which, as indicated in Chapter 5, include egg retrieval trauma to the bowel, appendix, bladder, and other organs; psychological effects like depression and high anxiety; and birth defects such as imprinting disorders (see later).

While adults can ask questions about the dangers of certain procedures or drugs, the fetus or child savior is generally passive. Dependent on the moral reasoning of his parents, he or she must cope with whatever dangers may crop up until he or she reaches the age of informed consent. When twentieth-century educational psychologist Jean Piaget researched intellectual development in children, he came up with a stages theory of cognitive development. The cognitive stage is crucial for informed consent and usually develops when a child is approximately 11 and thinks about individuals and abstract concepts like truth, morality, justice, and existence.

At this age children can judge the merits of savior donations to help others and can make adult decisions. Law professor Lois Weithorn's study to determine the age of consent in children (referred to in the *Cambridge Quarterly of Healthcare Ethics*, 2004) concluded that when children had to answer complex questions, the decision-making process of the 14-year-old was not much different from that of adult participants.

Medical procedures on minors or incompetents require informed consent, but if the parties cannot understand the consequences, a parent or guardian must give consent. If the court does not approve, this trumps the parent's decision. "Autonomy" is understood to mean self-determination, and in the medical context, respect for autonomy is what gives rise to the need for informed consent. In turn, informed consent requires that individuals are free from coercion and have access to reliable information. Since infants cannot give consent, they are due the moral right to adequate protection from harm from the courts.

The informed consent document should protect the patient and the healthcare provider; respect their autonomy and self-determination; touch on risks and benefits and claims of physician battery; and promote patient autonomy in safe and high-quality procedures, delivery of patient-centered medical care, and a workable patient-physician relationship. A doctor's failure to obtain the informed consent of his or her patient can subject the doctor to liability. Patients have brought legal action against fertility centers over claims of lack of informed consent; they allege they were not informed of the facility's lack of experience in performing PGD, the types of errors associated with PGD, or that they were not counseled about the option of performing PGD. Since informed consent often fails to communicate the risks and benefits, it is important that counselors intervene beforehand as a fail-safe measure to insure success.

Informed consent can vary in information packages—for example, there are formats such as a DVD, computer video, tutorial presentation, or computerized lessons. Some studies reveal the benefit of a multimedia approach such as Engaged MD, where the videos include information on controlled ovarian stimulation, embryo transfer, cryopreservation, and the health of an IVF baby. In a survey of 68 patients in April 2015, patients ranked Engaged MD second only to their doctor as an effective information source.

BEST INTEREST ETHIC

Informed consent of a minor, such as a savior donor, is only part of the legal infrastructure. Most courts also use the "best interest" standard regarding savior siblings. Under this philosophy a court determines whether allowing a child to donate tissue or organs would be in the best interests of the child and the child's needs. The court weighs the potential risks of the procedure against the benefits (*"Children's Anatomy v. Children's Autonomy," Pepperdine Law Review*, 2016). Often the court does not consider the wishes of the child but rather focuses more on the potential psychological benefits. Usually courts determine this by examining the siblings' relationship. If the siblings have a close relationship, the court will likely determine that the donor child would be better off psychologically in a normal family rather than in a family that suffered the death of a loved one. In these court cases the child's autonomy vies with the parents' right to reproduce and raise their children free from government intrusion.

The court usually applies the best interest standard. In the case of *Corran v. Bosze*, for example, the biological father of three-and-a-half-year-old twins asked the Illinois state court to compel the twins, against their mother's wishes, to donate bone marrow to their half brother who suffered from leukemia. The twins had met their stepbrother on only two occasions, each time lasting two hours. The court felt that a three-year-old has not yet developed the intent to become a bone marrow donor. The court held that a minor donor could undergo the procedure only when both parents give their informed consent and the procedure is in the best interest of the child.

The court mandated three factors: the parents must be informed of the risks and benefits, the parent who takes care of the child must be able to provide adequate emotional support, and a close existing relationship between the sick sibling and the donor sibling must exist. In the above case, the court decided the twins' mother would not be able to provide adequate support, the twins and the brother hardly knew each other, and surgery would not serve the twins' best interest.

SUBSTITUTED JUDGMENT STANDARD

Another standard that courts apply in savior cases was introduced in England in 1844 to guide guardians and courts in determining whether a formerly competent, now incompetent, individual could consent to a medical procedure. Known as the "substituted judgment standard," it directs primary caregivers in their actions since they would be imposing their belief on the patient's decision. In assessing whether a formerly competent individual would consent to a certain medical procedure, the caregiver must decide whether the individual ever expressed an intent regarding this type of medical treatment prior to becoming incompetent or indicated an intent based on his or her value system.

"EASY PGD": ONE POSSIBLE FUTURE

Earlier on in Chapter 1, the basics of PGD were laid out. Because of its ability to scan an eight-cell blastocyst to determine if the gene for a dangerous disease like Tay-Sachs is in the embryo, parents were able to choose to implant a safer embryo that would not only omit the disease gene but also conceive another child whose umbilical stem cells could help an older sibling or other relative.

The formula for "Easy PGD," as you probably guessed, grew out of the nuts and bolts of PGD. Although the science for safe and effective Easy PGD is likely to develop in the next 20–40 years, this is due to Easy PGD's production of many gametes. Greely predicts the elimination of the expense and discomfort of IVF, which now is a necessary prelude to PGD. Although at present it is the only relatively safe way to harvest oocytes, IVF is still a difficult process in which the woman typically has a 30–40 percent chance of success. Also, egg harvesting carries with it risks, such as loss of reproductive abilities, hospitalization, and death.

Easy PGD depends on the production of oocytes from skin cells. It also relates to sequencing the human genome and scanning for other diseases. The cost of sequencing the human genome has dropped from $500 million in 2003 to $1,000 in 2017. Genetics probably will continue to advance in this way and allow professionals to do cheap, accurate, and fast sequencing of the entire 6.4 billion base pair genome of an embryo.

GREELY'S FUTURE OF SAVIOR SIBLINGS

The above scenario presupposes future research into stem cell when skin cells will be tweaked into safe and effective gametes. Older women whose oocytes are losing potency will support this technique, and as the age of motherhood continues to rise, particularly women with higher education and income levels will help to encourage a healthy market for stem cell–derived eggs that could be fertilized in the laboratory with male sperm.

In an e-mail interview with Henry T. Greely, he explained that savior siblings would play a diminished role in a future of manufactured gametes, 100 embryos, and compatible HLAs. Greely envisions a time in which women will not have to undergo IVF hormone therapy and have eggs harvested to produce embryos for testing. That is because Easy PGD assumes that we will make major advances in the use of pluripotent stem cells (cells modified to form many cell types). Instead of conceiving a healthy child through IVF and PGD, the health professional could, instead, just take skin cells from the patient (with a genetically caused illness) and change them to make the person well. The protocol would be (a) select one of the 100 embryos made from skin cells with an HLA match that did not have the same predisposition for the genetic illness and (b) implant it in the mother's uterus.

Egg retrieval accounts for about 80 percent or more of the cost of IVF, most of the discomfort, and all the health risk. The good news is that PGD has not led to miscarriages, stillbirths, or neonatal deaths. Neither has it led to the births of babies missing large parts of their bodies. Greely infers that Easy PGD also will not lead to dangerous repercussions, and he approximates a cost of $11,000 for 100 embryos, which then could be analyzed for appropriateness as savior siblings.

PGD is the only abortion-free fetal diagnostic process, and considering that more than 6,000 single gene disorders can affect approximately one in 300 live births, the medical significance of Easy PGD is significant. (Easy PGD will not require FDA approval, but some of the sequencing methods will require FDA-reviewed devices.) If the technology of PGD continues to be effective, Greely predicts that 90 percent of the pregnant population would opt for it and for good reason: clinic staff would discriminate between healthy and bad embryos and would reject embryos that would not be viable.

In short, Greely says Easy PGD would work for savior siblings (100 embryos probably would be reduced to 25 HLA matching embryos), but in most cases, the lab worker would tweak new cells from the patient and make them into human embryonic stem cells without an autosomal recessive disease and transplant them (as you would stem cells from a savior sibling's umbilical cord).

Already in October 2016 a team of Japanese researchers, who pulled together accumulated research from around the world, took skin cells from mice and produced a batch of fertile offspring. How did they do it? The team reprogrammed the skin cells into stem cells and then into primordial germ cells that developed into mature eggs in a petri dish. Then they were fertilized in vitro and then implanted into adult mice that produced a new generation of pups.

Another way to produce eggs would be for a doctor to laparoscopically slice a bit of tissue from a woman's ovary and ripen the thousands of eggs in that tissue outside the woman's body. The advantage of taking and freezing ovarian slices in this surgical procedure would be that it is a one-time thing, and a woman would have more eggs than she could ever want.

Easy PGD would pave the way for more widespread use of this technique to treat individuals who cannot produce functional gametes. It also would prevent the birth of children who would suffer from incurable early onset diseases. Parents would get information regarding less worrisome gene-related health risks, such as a higher than average risk of coronary artery disease, type 1 diabetes, lupus, or colon cancer. Lastly PGD would be used to determine aesthetics such as hair, eye, and skin color; nose shape; hair type; height; the probability of male pattern baldness or early gray hair; and information on behavior such as intelligence, musical ability, sports strength, and mathematical talent.

Counselors would have to help parents with the interpretations of these 100 or so embryos, whose characteristics would be outlined on printouts, but once Easy PGD becomes popular, savior siblings will gradually fade out of use. Rather than birthing children whose purpose would be to serve as organ donors, the global community might encourage parents to use Easy PGD and HLA matching to avoid conceiving children with serious genetic ailments. If the obstetrician found the child to be genetically impaired in vivo, parents would then have the option of aborting this embryo. Parents would have greater control over the health of their children before conception.

Counselors would have to clarify to parents that just because they used Easy PGD, it does not mean their child will never become ill from genetic ailments. Counselors would have to emphasize that the technology only screens for a limited range of genetic features, and parents cannot expect to have a child free of every negative.

Greely believes that insurance companies will get behind this new technology of Easy PGD because they would end up paying less money in the long run if parents birthed children who had severe genetic ailments. Using ethical concepts such as fairness, justice, and equality, Greely predicts that the government would not interfere with Easy PGD except in an extreme instance—for instance, when a parent would select an embryo with a debilitating disease.

CONCLUSION

The reproductive world at 2050 will look quite different from what it is today, judging by experts such as Henry T. Greely. There may be a greater consolidation among fertility clinics, more discounts for individuals, and more sharing of innovative techniques.

Savior siblings and IVF may not be necessary what with Easy PGD and the creation of stem cells that can be tweaked into gametes. Although many people fear that the ethical restructuring from futuristic devices such as artificial wombs, 3D printed ovaries, and ovarian transplants will open the door to eugenics and human reproductive cloning, others are excited about the progress and opportunities for better health that tomorrow's ART will give birth to.

PART III

Scenarios

Case Studies

CASE STUDY I: CLARISSE AND BOB CANNOT AFFORD ART

Clarisse and Bob Fletcher feel despondent after visiting the fertility doctor. Although they are upper middle class with well-paying jobs, health insurance, and a house in the suburbs, they are not living the American dream. The fertility doctor says their ages (late 30s) are a negative, but he cannot pinpoint the exact cause of their inability to conceive. Unexplained infertility is the diagnosis. This usually indicates poor egg or sperm quality or problems with the uterus or fallopian tubes that are not identifiable during normal fertility testing. Clarisse and Bob prefer to believe they both have fertility problems, which makes the situation more tolerable.

Clarisse's doctor recommends IVF—he feels that since Clarisse is nearing age 40, she should skip artificial insemination. They know IVF is expensive and will probably need to be repeated several times. Everyday expenses are high since they have a mortgage and car payments, and their private health insurance does not cover expensive IVF treatments, which can range from $10,000 to $20,000. They wonder if they should give up their dream of having children or put a second mortgage on their house or borrow from their relatives until one IVF cycle works. On the first go-around, the doctor harvests six oocytes. They are fertilized with Bob's sperm, but only three embryos look healthy and the two transferred ones don't implant.

They next decide to get a loan from their bank, but the second IVF procedure also fails. One night on the TV news Bob hears a story about medical tourism and wonders if this might be their solution for lower-priced ART. Bob decides to do a Google search and look for clinics in Latin America. Terrorism and political tensions have discouraged them from traveling to Europe or Asia, so they search websites using the words "fertility tourism" and "South America." Neither of them has ever traveled abroad, so they are overwhelmed when they see the large number of clinics in Argentina, Brazil, Colombia, and Costa Rica. But pretty soon they are surfing from website to website and reading about the physicians, the procedures, and the lower prices.

Although these websites appear professional and well-staffed, Clarisse and Bob notice the frequent mention of one Argentine fertility clinic. They are impressed by the website's upbeat look, the detailed information, the highly trained health workers, and the glowing testimonials from past clients. They check out airfares and find they are affordable. They even track down an American couple who belongs to their baby support group and used the Argentine clinic. They volunteered some helpful feedback and smart tips.

Clarisse and Bob now feel better about going to a foreign clinic because the other couple assures them that everything is done competently, cautiously, and with great compassion. Clinic personnel can arrange flights and airport transfers, visas, accommodations, and interpreters. Clarisse asks about success rates, clinic staff expertise, and whether there are hidden costs. She is happy with the specifics she hears, especially that the couple's IVF produced a pregnancy, and they now have a baby girl.

Clarisse and Bob decide medical tourism is an option for them. Everything is so much more economical that they will be able to afford several IVF cycles. It doesn't hurt that both took Spanish in college, so they feel comfortable with the language although they are not fluent.

Despite their misgivings about safety and legal issues, Clarisse and Bob arrange to coordinate their spring vacations with the Argentina IVF trip, and they read everything they can get their hands on about the clinic and medical tourism in general. They are met at the airport by a concierge, who accompanies them to the clinic so Clarisse can have a physical exam and meet the doctor who will be harvesting her oocytes tomorrow. She already has been receiving hyperstimulating hormone shots, so her body is ready.

Unfortunately the hormone shots have increased her anxiety, and she is depending on the clinic personnel and Bob to calm her. That evening she takes a warm bath, meditates for 20 minutes, and then eats a healthy meal at her hotel. She tries to keep an optimistic attitude, and the relaxing music throughout the hotel helps to lull her into a state of contentment. This time, she tells herself, everything will work out the way it's supposed to.

Analysis

According to their fertility doctor, Clarisse and Bob may be in that 20 percent of infertile couples in which both partners have fertility problems. As noted in Chapter 1, women under 35 have more than a 40 percent chance of getting pregnant from IVF while women over 40 have only a

15 percent chance. Those who are 39 (like Clarisse) are statistically at the lower end.

Also, IVF cost is a big problem if you don't live in one of the 15 states that provide an insurance mandate or have top-flight employment insurance. Opportunities on the Internet to enter contests for free IVF cycles are tempting. You usually must tape a video and the clinic chooses a needy couple. Examples include the Sher Clinic in Las Vegas, the Red Rock Fertility in Las Vegas, and the Northern California Fertility Medical Clinic in Sacramento. But winning seems like a long shot, and taking out loans is a fast way to the poor house. Other American organizations, such as the Institute for Human Reproduction in Chicago, donate to people with meager finances.

Actually, medical tourism for IVF is less of a gamble than charities. Compared to the $18,000–$20,000 for IVF in the United States, Argentina, for instance, is a bargain, costing $4,300 for IVF, $4,700 for egg freezing, and $6,900 for egg donation. PGD is $500.

As discussed in Chapter 2, there are over 3,000 fertility clinics around the world, including over 500 in India alone and over 200 in Spain. Couples can comparison shop and choose the most economical and convenient geographical area.

CASE STUDY 2: GABE NEEDS A SAVIOR

Laura and Phil Johnson are in their 30s and never thought they would be in their present predicament. If their two-year-old son Gabe is to live a healthy, normal life, he needs a miracle in the form of a sibling with no genetic diseases. Doctors advise the couple to give birth to a savior sibling for their son, who has recently been diagnosed with thalassemia. Thalassemia is a recessive blood disorder caused by mutations in a gene located on chromosome 11. Children like Gabe, who inherit both mutations of thalassemia, usually have severe anemia requiring lifelong treatment with blood transfusions to maintain satisfactory levels of hemoglobin. They also need iron-chelation therapy to combat iron overload in the body. Both treatments are dangerous. Without treatment, affected patients like Gabe have shortened life expectancies, and regular transfusion programs extend life expectancy only until the individual reaches his 30s–50s.

However, with a transfusion of stem cells from a matched donor, Gabe can be cured of his condition. But, since Gabe currently has no close relatives that are a genetic match, a donor, in the form of a sibling, would have to be engineered. Laura and Phil are both carriers for thalassemia, so the odds are high that they could produce a second child with thalassemia if they do not combine ART with PGD to get the best fertilized embryo match. Laura and Phil feel they are between a rock and a hard place and are overwhelmed by the responsibility. The couple wanted another child but not under these life-and-death circumstances. They feel enormous pressure and have a lot of questions: What if they cannot produce the right oocytes or sperm? What if the gametes turn out to be carriers of other genetic diseases? Can Gabe survive until the doctors can transplant just the right fertilized embryo? Is PGD so perfect that a biopsied embryo that passes muster can work a miracle for Gabe? Would they be better off to let nature take its course and let Gabe struggle with his disease without involving another child?

The ethical dilemma is difficult. The couple knows they cannot live with the guilt of not doing everything possible to save Gabe even if it's at the expense of a new baby, but they also know the "savior" child must be treasured and not viewed as only a resource. The couple has been briefed about savior siblings from their doctor and has read the Jodi Picoult book *My Sister's Keeper*. Despite this preparation and the encouragement of family and friends, they have mixed feelings about conceiving a child as a donor even though they know they will love this child unconditionally. Still they worry. What if the new child comes to resent the circumstances under which he or she was conceived?

Mainly, though, they cannot bear the thought of losing Gabe. No other therapy will give Gabe a fighting chance, and they comfort themselves with the thought that the therapy will not be invasive—doctors will take stem cells from the new sibling's umbilical cord blood and inject them into Gabe's circulatory system.

Everyone in their family has a different opinion. Gabe's grandparents are in denial and say to wait and that maybe the disease won't be as bad as the doctors think. Their friends are excited over this twenty-first-century high-tech fertility process and are curious to see what will happen. And Laura and Phil love Gabe and are invested emotionally in his welfare and future health.

Naturally Laura and Phil did a lot of Internet research before initiating another pregnancy. They read how an Arab couple had a similar situation. They produced four healthy embryos of which one was a match. As soon as the child was old enough to understand, the couple explained the younger son's importance to the older one. The bond deepened between the two boys and brought the family closer. Laura and Phil hope they follow in the footsteps of this family and heal Gabe while building a healthy future with their two children.

Analysis

A savior child guarantees that the affected child will have a disease-free survival rate of over 90 percent, and as noted in Chapter 7, most religions allow IVF and PGD in genetic disease cases. That said, the ethics disturb many couples due to the genetic scanning and the discarding of a series of embryos before finding one without the disease gene and with a compatible HLA (Human Leukocyte Antigens).

As pointed out in Chapter 10, the ethics of savior child conception include parental autonomy, which confers on parents the right to decide for their child what is the best option. They want beneficence in maintaining the children's health and justice in ensuring that the unborn child has a good life. They also want to avoid placing a monetary burden on society for a cure the parents can provide.

Counselors say successful saviors develop great self-esteem, although anger, guilt, and blame affect "failing" saviors. Anxiety sometimes arises. As presented in Chapter 10, Cambridge University study researchers followed 198 families for seven years and found that donor IVF children had more emotional problems than natural-born children due to anxiety over high parental expectations.

Savior children also must cope with other challenges. Wendy Pack of Pacific Graduate School of Psychology says the savior child may envy the attention his or her sibling receives as well as develop a low self-concept due to his or her unique birth. Some savior siblings who undergo multiple trips to the hospital sometimes lack a normal childhood. About one-third of savior siblings develop PTSD with guilt and inferiority.

Alternative programs can make a difference. Some families can locate donor genetic materials if there is standardization in umbilical cord banking, and they do genetic testing of parents before procreation. Another method is to combine the prophylactic use of IVF and PGD. Bioethicist Susan Wolf favors assigning the donor child to one doctor and insisting that harvesting be carried out only with the permission of parents and an ethics body. Besides counseling, art therapists and donor advocates can assist in the process, as suggested by the American Academy of Pediatrics.

CASE STUDY 3: DIANE AND SHELLY WANT A BIOLOGICAL CHILD

Although their sexual preferences have been well known since they were teenagers, Diane and Shelly, both now 35, worried that their lesbianism would interfere with their decision to conceive and parent a biological child. It was one thing to allow marriage between two consenting adults of the same sex, but it was another thing to introduce a biological child into the mix. Although studies indicate that children are not harmed having two "mommies," social values have not yet caught up with scientific research. Even doctors hesitated when they heard Diane and Shelly's story, and some refused to do IVF at all on a lesbian couple.

The plan was to use Diane's egg with a male friend as a sperm donor. They liked this donor because he was healthy, handsome, and honorable but did not want any responsibility for raising the child even though Diane and Shelly let him know that he was free to love the child as much as he desired. Despite the absence of any contract or legal papers, Diane and Shelly did not foresee any complications. Maybe they were naïve, but they figured that contracts and lawyers would be one more hassle, and Diane and Shelly worried that their male friend might back out.

Also, their fertility doctor was not happy with the couple's choice of male donor. He preferred washed sperm and complete anonymity. Diane tried four IUI cycles, which all failed. The fertility doctors thought that perhaps the donor sperm the couple insisted on using was working against them. "If it was going to happen this way, it would have already," the physicians said. Their reactions sounded biased and negative, but the two women decided to be proactive and ignore this discrimination.

So they registered at a clinic that specialized in same-sex couples. The doctors there recommended Shelly carry the pregnancy but since she was uncomfortable with the idea of a visible pregnancy—because she is a college professor—she declined.

Even at this more enlightened clinic, the doctors had difficulty equalizing their treatment of both partners. They hurt the couple's feelings several times by never using the adjective "our." It was never "our" baby, the two women complain. It was always "her" baby. Just because they didn't bring a man to the office, the doctor refused to speak to them together. He said his patient is the one undergoing IVF, not the female partner. Worse, the couple has had little access to support resources like donor egg counseling that heterosexual couples routinely get.

They are lucky that their ART procedures are covered by insurance whereas surrogacy is not. Surrogacy and using another woman's egg would be possible if it weren't so expensive and denied them the genetic link. The couple also would not be able to physically experience the birth. Adoption is always on the table, but that would mean giving up their wish to have a genetically related child.

The new doctors inform the women that they are both experiencing infertility; their eggs are older, and even if Shelley volunteers to take fertility drugs and produce a fertilized embryo, she might have as much difficulty as her partner has. Even if she gets pregnant, she may miscarry. They decide to take that approach anyway.

Diane and Shelly know they are not alone in their desire since there are lots of lesbians and homosexuals in their support group who are trying to get pregnant, but sometimes they cannot tolerate the bias. The discrimination is especially bad when the couple has to speak to the insurance assistant, who always asks to see Diane's "husband's" card.

The couple must reveal their infertility to their employers to take medical leave and visit doctors' offices, and although their families are supportive, more than one person questions their decision making and asks about finances and timing. Diane and Shelly resent having to justify their choice. Married heterosexual couples don't have to tolerate this level of scrutiny, they feel. The couple realizes they are in a cultural bind where social stigma has forced them to make public their sexual orientation. This will not reduce the quality of their parenting, however. Despite having to jump through hoops to show their understanding of this special family configuration, they intend to see it through with IVF because having a genetic child will help to solidify their marriage.

Analysis

Experts say about 200,000–1,000,000 same-sex couples wish to become genetic parents. IUI comes with a 20–24 percent success rate for women under age 35, and by age 40, success is only 10 percent per try. These statistics may help Diane and Shelly, but they still contribute to the discrimination and medicalization of LBGT reproduction, as pointed out in the *APA Newsletter*, spring 2016. The result is that clinics with their heterosexual mind-set treat lesbians as if they are automatically infertile. They recommend aggressive treatment protocols, portraying self-insemination (AI) as dangerous. Instead of encouraging IUI, they often recommend going directly to IVF.

Clinics also display homophobic reactions and moral judgments of lesbian motherhood despite the ASRM and APA reporting that children raised by single parents, gays, or lesbians are not harmed or disadvantaged. Healthcare workers sometimes irritate lesbian couples by presuming they want a child so they can feel more "normal." Research also shows that physicians in SART-affiliated clinics show a slightly higher number of accepted single heterosexual women than lesbian couples. One lesbian was told by her family practitioner to lie about her sexuality and bring a male friend along to her fertility appointment. As mentioned in Chapter 8, common objections to lesbian motherhood include a confused gender identity of the child, the stigma of having a lesbian parent, and the selfishness of desiring a child.

Online support groups and bulletin boards help bolster LBGTs. These resources include Parents, Families and Friends of Lesbians and Gays, the Lesbian and Gay Family Building Project in Western New York, Maybe Baby (Seattle), Los Angeles Gay Center's Family Services, Family Matters of San Diego, and Rainbow Families.

CASE STUDY 4: THE COHENS WANT A CHILD OF THE JEWISH FAITH

Abby and Mitchell Cohen, orthodox Jews in their early 40s, attend Rosh Hashanah services at their neighborhood synagogue. They watch the children romp and play tag and feel sad. The Cohens have been trying to become pregnant for five years. They wonder if they will ever fit into their religious community. They suffer most from feeling left out of certain religious rituals and celebrations.

While people usually show sympathy for parents having behavioral problems with children, those same people often do not offer any solace to couples undergoing ART procedures to conceive children. They figure it's none of their business, and since theological principles admonish Jews to be fruitful and multiply, temple members infer that childless couples have fertility problems. So, they don't want to bring up an uncomfortable topic. Some members are less than tactful, and Abby has had to put up with comments like "you're not getting pregnant because you're stressed" or "you're letting your career dictate your whole life." She does not reply to these remarks, but she secretly wonders if the infertility isn't her fault. Mitchell does not blame her, but sometimes she can tell he envies his brother, who has two small boys.

Conversations about children monopolize social events at the temple. Children participate in festivals like Purim and attend Sunday school where they learn Bible stories and songs. The temple general fund even pays for babysitters to mind children during Friday night services.

The Cohens especially feel distressed at Seders, where children ask "The Four Questions," a tradition that the youngest members enjoy. Once Abby was so overcome with sadness at a Bris (a circumcision ceremony) that she teared up while everyone else was smiling, laughing, and memorializing the occasion with wine and hors d'oeuvres. Her emotions were so raw that people must have thought she was mourning a child or parent who had recently died. Even celebrating weekly Shabbats is hard because of all the children playing games and telling riddles. Sometimes she wants to hug them, and other times, she feels like running out of the synagogue and retreating to her bedroom.

Abby and Mitchell, like many couples, do not acknowledge their infertility problem even to their families. Neither have they sought out emotional support from their rabbi. They are, however, receiving help from a fertility doctor and have undergone three IVF procedures, none of which worked.

To retain autonomy, Abby and Mitchell decide to give the daily shots at home. So instead of having to rush in and out of the clinic nurse's office, Abby can rest at home in privacy, using that time to relax and visualize herself and her husband in a favorite setting—for example, the field of Galilee beside a crystal-clear running river. She continues doing prayerful imagery and picturing the positive changes taking place within her body. She intends to try acupuncture too. One woman in Abby's online support group shares the practice of "Chana's Prayer," a prayer that women say when struggling with fertility.

The Cohens realize they are getting old even for IVF, so they agree to a plan B: adoption. Their support group has given them names of Jewish adoption organizations. Even if you cannot adopt a Jewish child, you can convert a child born from a non-Jewish mother. The process is easier for girls, but a little more complicated for boys. Boys must be circumcised by a mohel, immersed in rainwater in a mikveh, all under the supervision of a beit din, a group of three rabbinic authorities. Baby girls require the mikveh immersion and a Hebrew name. The Cohens feel that adoption would be a good choice if IVF does not yield results.

Another fallback plan is something that Abby is keeping to herself because she isn't sure she could go through with it. Her sister has offered to become a surrogate, using Mitchell's sperm. It is a generous gift, and genetically speaking, better than adoption, but Abby is not sure she can bear to have another woman—even her younger sister—carry her child. While this has the advantage of knowing the baby's genetic inheritance, Abby worries she will not be able to bond with a child who may seem more like a nephew or niece than a son or daughter. Abby intends to seek counsel from the rabbi before she broaches the subject to Mitchell.

Analysis

The Pew Forum surveyed American Jews in 2013 and found that Jewish adults aged 40–59 report having fewer children due to fertility problems—an average of 1.9 children compared with 2.2 children among the general American public. Fertility doctor Vincent Brandeis estimates that in 60 percent of his Orthodox Jewish patients, infertility is due to sperm quality, motility, and number. The top therapies for Jews are noted in Chapter 7. They are IVF, surrogacy, and adoption.

According to the Jewish website Kveller, IVF contradicts Jewish law because it leads to unused fertilized eggs. However, Jewish authorities say eggs fertilized outside the womb do not have any human status and can be discarded. And selective reduction can be overcome, says Rabbi Elliot Dorff, by limiting implantation to two or three embryos to avoid abortion.

Decision making is difficult, but help can come from online infertility resources like T.I.M.E. (A Torah Infertility Medium of Exchange), the Jewish organization Hasidah, the column "The Practical Rabbi" by Rabbi Michael Gold, and the book *And Hannah Wept: Infertility, Adoption and the Jewish Couple*.

The option of surrogacy, according to most Orthodox and Conservative rabbis, is permitted, but the Jewish status of the child is determined not by the child's genetic material but by the mother who carries the child to term. Rabbis require conversion for any child born to a non-Jewish surrogate.

As for adoption, the percentage of nonwhite children adopted into Jewish families has steadily increased; of children adopted between 2000 and 2012, 34 percent were white, 32 percent were Asian or Asian-mixed, 17 percent were Latino or Latino-mixed, and 15 percent were black or black-mixed. Resources for adoption include the Jewish Children's Adoption Network, Jewish Child and Family Service, and the Jewish Foster and Adoption Network.

CASE STUDY 5: THE CLARKS WANT A SECOND FAMILY

When Joyce and Alan Clark were in their 20s, they married their college sweethearts and had two children each. They then divorced. Now at age 39 and remarried, they would like to have a child related to both. But they are having fertility problems. Alan's sperm count has diminished, and Joyce may not be ovulating each month as her menstrual periods are erratic. While taking the combined oral contraceptive pill, she also became hypertensive. Now, off the pill, she still has mild hypertension controlled by medication. Her hypertension works against fertility and carrying a child to full term.

Even so, Joyce and Alan want to try fertility treatments because they believe their four teenagers will bond faster if they can anticipate a new addition to the family. Of course, jealousy might erupt, but they think that it is something that can be handled with family counseling and common sense. Joyce is a high school teacher and knows that role modeling appropriate behavior will go a long way toward demonstrating to the teenagers that babies are not only a lot of work but also exciting and joyful. Besides, the child will share the genetic traits of everyone in the family and that should help unify everyone.

The fertility doctor advises IVF since Joyce and Alan have been trying to get pregnant naturally for over a year. So, Joyce takes hormonal medications to induce ovulation and suffers some milder symptoms of OHSS (ovarian hyperstimulation syndrome), such as mood swings and bloating. She tries not to complain too much because the emotional challenge of relating well to four teenagers is her priority. So, if anyone asks how she is feeling, she says "fine."

Joyce would like to have a multiple pregnancy to save money and time. She has read about celebrities with twin IVF babies and thinks this would be great fun for her and Alan. A single embryo transplant, which her doctor recommends, seems too conservative. She has been reading scientific studies on the Internet, and not everyone agrees with her physician. She could switch doctors and find someone to implant two embryos, but she has built a certain trust with her current doctor and doesn't feel much like delaying things until she finds another physician.

The couple also is anxious over the costs of IVF and the additional expense of a new infant. They have decent salaries, and the teens have trust funds set up by their grandparents, but they also will need extra money for college extras like airfare and computers. The teens want to get part-time jobs because all their friends are doing it, but Joyce and Alan would rather have them concentrate on school.

Joyce and Alan feel the more time the teens spend with the baby now, the better the stepfamily relationship will be. The couple knows that teens like to socialize with their peers, but Joyce hopes to convince them to spend some quality time with the new baby because in a few years they will be off to college and careers and won't have the opportunity to get to know and appreciate the newest member of the family.

Joyce and Alan also are not getting emotional support from parents and in-laws. Their relatives think they should skip building a second family. They say it will cause a strain in the marriage, and they've already been through one divorce—they certainly don't want to go through another. Joyce's mother thinks she has too much on her plate—a job, four teens, a new husband, and now these IVF trials. But Alan is very supportive, so Joyce is not as worried as she might be. She is more worried about gaining weight. The last time she saw her doctor he mentioned that obesity works against pregnancy. With high blood pressure, she doesn't need extra pounds.

When she gets anxious, she eats and then gets angry at herself for sabotaging her health. She'd like to be calmer, but her temperament is not always easy to manage. Perhaps she should take her colleague's advice and sign up for a night class in mind-body control or biofeedback. The techniques might relax her and get her mind off her infertility problems.

Analysis

Controversy surrounds the definition of what is the "right" number of implanted embryos. A *Reproductive BioMedicine* (Bissonnette et al., 2011) study transferred one embryo in half the cases and two or more in the rest; the pregnancy rate was 32 percent for the single group compared with 42 percent for the multiple method.

This is no surprise to Medical Director Norbert Gleicher at the Center for Human Reproduction of New York City. He says IVF patients are closely monitored and face fewer risks. In a 2014 paper in *Fertility and Sterility* he argued that two singleton pregnancies carry the same risk as one twin pregnancy, and PGD helps doctors select healthy embryos to transfer.

But twin pregnancies don't always go well. As discussed in Chapter 5, risks include low birth weight, prematurity, and prolonged hospitalization. The birth mother also encounters risks. Moreover, the average cost of a twin pregnancy is four times that of a singleton. Health journalist Jane Brody says clinics often suggest transplanting multiple embryos to increase their "success" rate.

According to a Cochrane report, hypertension medications like the one Joyce takes carry some risks such as preterm labor, gestational diabetes, and babies with cerebral palsy and learning disabilities. Some doctors stop the medications if the hypertension is mild.

Adding a biological child to the mix will probably stir up insecurities, says the website parenting.com, but it often gives the stepparent relationship solidarity and confidence. As noted in Chapter 6, some kids may react with jealousy, anxiety, or excitement, but the best parenting strategy is to listen patiently to all objections and resentments.

Family counseling may be a smart strategy. The U.S. Bureau of Census (2006) reports that second marriages with or without children have a 60 percent rate of divorce, and long-term studies find that remarriage is more difficult than divorce. So along with counseling, it's best to involve the children in the planning of the new baby, get their input on names, and help them feel part of the process.

GLOSSARY

Achondroplasia: Hereditary condition resulting in very short limbs and sometimes a face that is small in relation to the (normal-sized) skull.

Amenorrhea: A condition in which a woman doesn't have menstrual periods.

Antisperm Antibody Test: A test that can determine if antibodies on the surface of sperm are interfering with the ability of sperm to move, penetrate the cervical mucus, or fertilize an egg.

ART (Assisted Reproductive Technology): All treatments or procedures that include the in vitro handling of both human oocytes and sperm or embryos to establish a pregnancy. Includes but is not limited to in vitro fertilization and embryo transfer, gamete intrafallopian transfer, zygote intrafallopian transfer, tubal embryo transfer, gamete and embryo cryopreservation, oocyte and embryo donation, and gestational surrogacy. ART does not include assisted insemination (artificial insemination), which uses sperm from either a woman's partner or a sperm donor.

Artificial insemination: The general name for the procedure in which sperm are inserted directly into a woman's cervix, tubes, or uterus.

ASRM: The American Society for Reproductive Medicine, a nonprofit dedicated to reproductive medicine with an affiliate called SART, the Society for Assisted Reproductive Technologies.

Assisted hatching: A form of ART when an embryologist uses micromanipulation under a microscope to create a small hole in the zona pellucida of the egg.

Azoospermia: When a man has no sperm present in his semen.

Biochemical pregnancy (preclinical spontaneous abortion/miscarriage): A pregnancy diagnosed only by the detection of HCG in serum or urine and that does not develop into a clinical pregnancy.

Blastocyst: A human embryo from the fifth day after fertilization until implantation.

Cancelled cycle: An ART cycle in which ovarian stimulation or monitoring has been carried out with the intention to treat but did not proceed to follicular aspiration or, in the case of a thawed embryo, to embryo transfer.

Chorionic villi sampling: A form of prenatal diagnosis to determine chromosomal or genetic disorders in the fetus.

Clinical pregnancy: A pregnancy diagnosed by ultrasonographic visualization of one or more gestational sacs or definitive clinical signs of pregnancy. Includes ectopic pregnancy.

Clomid: A fertility drug given to women to stimulate ovulation.

Clone: An exact copy of something with the same DNA, sometimes produced through somatic cell nuclear transfer.

Congenital anomalies: All structural, functional, and genetic anomalies diagnosed in aborted fetuses, at birth, or in the neonatal period.

Controlled ovarian stimulation: Pharmacological treatment in which women are stimulated to induce the development of multiple ovarian follicles to obtain multiple oocytes at follicular aspiration.

Cryopreservation: Freezing of a specimen, either semen or embryos, such as in liquid nitrogen (−196 degrees C) to keep embryos viable to store them for future transfer into a uterus or to keep sperm viable for future insemination or ART procedures.

Delivery: The expulsion or extraction of one or more fetuses from the mother after 20 completed weeks of gestational age.

Donor eggs: The eggs taken from the ovaries of a fertile woman and donated to an infertile woman to be used in an ART procedure.

Donor embryo transfer: The transfer of embryos resulting from the oocyte (egg) and sperm of another patient, who may be anonymous or known, to an otherwise infertile recipient.

Down syndrome: A genetic disorder caused by the presence of an extra chromosome 21 and characterized by mental retardation, abnormal facial features, and medical problems such as heart defects.

Ectopic pregnancy: A pregnancy outside the uterus, the fallopian tube being the most common site.

Egg retrieval: The procedure of harvesting oocytes (eggs) by a minimally invasive surgical procedure during an IVF cycle. This is done under light anesthesia so that patients are asleep. Typically takes about 30 minutes total.

Eggs: The female sex cells (ova) produced by the female's ovaries, which, when fertilized by a male's sperm, produce embryos, the early form of human life.

Elective embryo transfer: The transfer of one or more embryos selected from a larger cohort of available embryos.

Embryo: The earliest developmental stage of an organism. In humans it begins with the fertilization of the egg and lasts until the end of the eighth week after fertilization, when it is renamed as a fetus.

Embryo donation: The transfer of an embryo resulting from gametes (sperm and oocytes) that do not originate from the recipient and her partner.

Embryo/fetus reduction: A procedure to reduce the number of viable embryos or fetuses in a multiple pregnancy.

Embryo transfer: Placement of an embryo into the uterus through the vagina and cervix or, in the case of zygote intrafallopian transfer (ZIFT) or tubal embryo transfer (TET), into the fallopian tube.

Endometriosis: The presence of endometrial tissue (tissue that normally lines the uterus) in abnormal locations such as the ovaries, fallopian tubes, and abdominal cavity. These lesions lead to local irritation and inflammation that can cause scarring that can impede pelvic organs to the point of dysfunction and pain.

Endometrium: The lining of the uterus that is shed each month with the menstrual period. The endometrium thickens and thus provides a nourishing site for the implantation of a fertilized egg.

Estradiol: The predominant estrogen (hormone) produced by the follicular cells of the ovary.

FDA: The Food and Drug Administration, which in the United States regulates drugs, medical devices, and biological products.

Fertilization: The penetration of the ovum by the sperm and combination of their genetic material resulting in the formation of a zygote.

Fetal death (stillbirth): Death prior to the complete expulsion or extraction from its mother of a product of fertilization, at or after 20 completed weeks of gestational age. The death is indicated by fetus not breathing or showing any other evidence of life such as heartbeat, umbilical cord pulsation, or definite movement of voluntary muscles.

Fetus: An unborn child.

Fibroid: A benign tumor of muscular and fibrous tissues, typically developing in the wall of the uterus.

Follicle-stimulating hormone (FSH): In women, FSH is the pituitary hormone responsible for stimulating follicular cells in the ovary to grow, stimulating egg development and the production of the female hormone estrogen. In the male, FSH helps travel through the bloodstream to the testes and helps stimulate them to manufacture sperm. FSH also can be given as a medication.

Frozen-thawed embryo transfer cycle: An ART procedure in which cycle monitoring is carried out with the intention of transferring frozen-thawed embryos.

Full-term birth: A live birth or stillbirth that takes place between 37 and 42 completed weeks of gestational age.

Gamete: A mature germ cell (egg or sperm) able to unite with a gamete from the other sex to form a zygote.

Gamete intrafallopian transfer (GIFT): An ART procedure in which both gametes (oocytes and spermatozoa) are transferred to the fallopian tube.

Gestational carrier (surrogate): A woman who carries an embryo to delivery. The embryo is derived from the egg and sperm of persons not related to the carrier. The carrier has no genetic relationship with the resulting child.

Gonadotropin-releasing hormone (GnRH): A hormone produced in the hypothalamus of the brain that is involved in triggering ovulation. Sold under the name Factrel and Lutrepulse.

Hepatitis B and C: Viruses that may be sexually transmitted or transmitted by contact with blood and other bodily fluids that can cause infection of the liver leading to jaundice and liver failure.

High-order multiple: A pregnancy or delivery with three or more fetuses or neonates.

Human chorionic gonadotropin (HCG): A hormone that increases early in pregnancy. This hormone is produced by the placenta; its detection is the basis of most pregnancy tests. It also can be used as a luteinizing hormone (LH) substitute to trigger ovulation in conjunction with clomiphene or gonadotropin therapy. Sold under the names Novarel, Pregnyl, and Ovidrel.

Human immunodeficiency virus (HIV): A retrovirus that causes acquired immune deficiency syndrome (AIDS), a disease that destroys the body's ability to protect itself from infection and disease. It is transmitted by the exchange of bodily fluids or blood transfusions.

Hysterosalpinogram (HSG): An X-ray procedure in which a special media (a dye-like solution) is injected through the cervix into the uterine cavity to show the inner shape of the uterus and degree of openness of the fallopian tubes.

Hysteroscopy: The insertion of a long, thin, lighted telescope-like instrument through the cervix and into the uterus to examine the inside of the uterus.

Implantation: The attachment and subsequent penetration by the zona-free blastocyst that starts five to seven days after fertilization.

In vitro fertilization (IVF): An assisted reproduction technique where egg and sperm are united outside a woman's body to form a zygote and embryo, which is then transferred into a woman's uterus for implantation and pregnancy.

Infertility: A disease of the reproductive system defined by the failure to achieve a clinical pregnancy after 12 months or more of regular unprotected sexual intercourse.

Initiated cycle: An ART cycle in which the woman received specific medication for ovarian stimulation or monitoring in the case of natural cycles with the intention to treat.

Intracytoplasmic sperm injection (ICSI): An assisted reproduction technique where a single sperm will be injected directly into an egg, initiating fertilization.

Intrauterine insemination (IUI): An artificial insemination technique in which sperm are put directly into a woman's uterus at the time she is ovulating.

Laparoscope/laparoscopic surgery: A thin, lighted viewing instrument with a telescopic lens through which a surgeon views the exterior surfaces of a female's reproductive organs and abdominal cavity. The laparoscope is placed through the belly button to view and operate on the abdominal cavity and reproductive organs.

Medically assisted reproduction: Brought about through ovulation induction, controlled ovarian stimulation, ovulation triggering ART procedures, and intra-uterine, intracervical, and intravaginal insemination with semen of a husband/partner or a donor.

Mild ovarian stimulation for IVF: A procedure in which the ovaries are stimulated with gonadotropins and/or other compounds, with the intent to limit the number of oocytes obtained for IVF to fewer than seven.

Mitochondrial DNA: DNA found in one circular chromosome inside the mito-chondrion. In humans this DNA has about 16,600 base pairs and codes for about 37 genes.

Modified natural cycle: An IVF procedure in which one or more oocytes are collected from the ovaries during a spontaneous menstrual cycle. Drugs are administered with the sole purpose of blocking the spontaneous LH surge and/or inducing final oocyte maturation.

Morphology: The size and shape of sperm.

Mosaicism: An organism that has more than one version of a genome, all derived from the same zygote, or fertilized egg.

Motility: The ability of sperm to move by themselves.

Natural cycle IVF: An IVF procedure in which one or more oocytes are collected from the ovaries during a spontaneous menstrual cycle without any drug use.

Ovarian hyperstimulation syndrome (OHSS): An exaggerated systemic response to ovarian stimulation characterized by a wide spectrum of clinical and laboratory symptoms. It is classified as mild, moderate, or severe according to the degree of abdominal distention, ovarian enlargement, and respiratory, hemodynamic, and metabolic complications.

Ovarian torsion: The partial or complete rotation of the ovarian vascular pedicle that causes obstruction to ovarian blood flow, potentially leading to necrosis of ovarian tissue.

Ovulation: The release of a mature egg from its developing follicle in the outer layer of the ovary. This usually occurs approximately 14 days preceding the next menstrual period.

Ovulation induction: The administration of hormone medications (ovulation drugs) that stimulate the ovaries to ovulate.

Pelvic inflammatory disease: Inflammation of the uterus, fallopian tubes, and ovaries due to infection and sometimes a cause of infertility in women.

Polycystic ovary syndrome: A common endocrine condition that causes hormonal imbalances in women of reproductive age. It can lead to dysfunctional ovulation, infertility, weight gain, prediabetes, and an increase in the male hormone, testosterone.

Preimplantation genetic diagnosis (PGD): The process of doing genetic testing on one or more cells from an embryo for determining the likely traits of those embryos to decide which embryos to transfer for possible implantation and birth.

Preimplantation genetic screening (PGS): Analysis of polar bodies, blastomeres, or trophectoderm from oocytes, zygotes, or embryos for the detection of aneuploidy, mutation, and/or DNA rearrangement.

Premature ovarian failure: A condition in which a woman enters menopause before age 40, with the ovaries ceasing ovulation and the production of estrogen.

Progesterone: A female hormone secreted by the corpus luteum after ovulation during the second half of the menstrual cycle. It prepares the lining of the uterus for implantation of a fertilized egg and allows for complete shedding of the endometrium at the time of menstruation.

Semen analysis: The microscopic examination of semen to determine the number of sperm, their shapes, and their ability to move.

Sperm: The male reproductive cells that fertilize a woman's egg. The sperm head carries genetic material; the midpiece produces energy for movement; and the long, thin tail wiggles to propel the sperm.

Spontaneous abortion/miscarriage: The spontaneous loss of a clinical pregnancy that occurs before 20 completed weeks of gestational age.

Surrogacy: In traditional surrogacy, a woman is inseminated with the sperm of a man who is not her partner to conceive and carry a child to be reared by the biological (genetic) father and his partner. In this procedure the surrogate is genetically related to the child. The biological father and his partner must usually adopt the child after his or her birth. Another type of surrogate is a gestation carrier, a woman who is implanted with the fertilized embryo of another couple to carry the pregnancy. The surrogate is not genetically related to the child in this case.

Thalassemia: Any of a group of hereditary hemolytic diseases caused by faulty hemoglobin synthesis.

Transvaginal ultrasound aspiration: An ultrasound-guided technique for egg retrieval. A long, thin needle is passed through the vagina into the ovarian follicle, and suction is applied to retrieve the egg. Also known as ultrasound-guided egg aspiration and transvaginal egg retrieval.

Uterus: The hollow, muscular organ in the pelvis where an embryo implants and grows during pregnancy. The lining of the uterus, called the endometrium, produces the monthly menstrual blood flow when there is no pregnancy.

Varicocele: A varicose vein around the ductus (vas) deferens and the testes. This may be a cause of low sperm counts, motility, and morphology and may lead to male infertility.

Vitrification: An ultrarapid cryopreservation method that prevents ice formation within the suspension, which is converted to a glass-like solid.

Zona pellucida: The thick transparent membrane surrounding an ovum before implantation.

Zygote: A fertilized egg.

Zygote intrafallopian transfer (ZIFT): Oocytes (eggs) are aspirated, fertilized in the laboratory, and surgically transferred into the fallopian tubes before cell division. This procedure has largely been replaced by IVF.

Source: Adapted from "Third-Party Reproduction: A Guide for Patients," Patient Information Series, ASRM, 2012; World Health Organization (WHO) Revised Glossary on ART Terminology, 2009; and WebMD Medical Reference, December 2016.

TIMELINE

3 CE   Records show Jewish thinkers discussed the possibility of human insemination by artificial means.

1677   Sperm first viewed under a microscope.

1777   An Italian priest conducts experiments with artificial insemination in reptiles.

1790   First successful case of human artificial insemination (AI) is reported by Scottish surgeon John Hunter.

1827   Early research in which scientists first learn that the female body contains eggs called ova.

1843   Scientists discover that conception takes place when a sperm from the male reproductive system enters an ovum.

1855   The Woman's Hospital opens in New York, and chief doctor J. Marion Sims believes that most infertility can be cured through gynecological surgery. But he agrees to perform AI in those women who refuse surgical methods. Fifty-five times over a two-year period Sims injects a husband's sperm into his wife's uterus, but his experiments result in only one pregnancy that ends in miscarriage.

1873   The book *Sex in Education* by Harvard doctor Edward Clarke argues that having a college education contributes to sterility among young women.

1876   As the field of medicine is increasingly professionalized, the American Gynecological Society is formed; J. Marion Sims is one of its founders.

1884   First successful case of U.S. human donor insemination by physician William Pancoast at the Jefferson Medical College in Philadelphia.

He injects sperm from a medical student into an anesthetized woman. She gives birth to a boy nine months later. Pancoast never tells the woman what he has done and only shares the information with her husband several years later.

1890   Future infertility doctor John Rock is born in Massachusetts.

1901   Hans Spemann splits a two-celled newt embryo into two parts, successfully producing two larvae.

1906   Surgeon Robert Tuttle Morris, who has been conducting partial ovarian transplantations from healthy women to those unable to have children, witnesses the first (and only) successful pregnancy in a recipient.

1909   When an account of Pancoast's actions involving AI by donor appears in the *Medical World* journal 25 years after it took place, the doctor is strongly criticized.

1909   Future IVF researcher Landrum Brewer Shettles is born.

1910   Howard Jones is born. His work with wife Georgeanna in the field of IVF will lead to America's first "test tube baby."

Former president Theodore Roosevelt declares, "The greatest of all curses is the curse of sterility; and severest of all condemnation should be ... visited upon willful sterility."

1912   Future IVF pioneer Georgeanna Jones is born.

1917   John Del-Zio with his wife will become the first American couple to seek IVF treatment.

1922   Principally funded by the Rockefeller Foundation, the Committee for Research in Problems of Sex is founded and spends much of the next 20 years supporting research in the field of reproductive endocrinology (the study of reproductive hormones) as well as in the field of human sexuality research of Dr. Alfred Kinsey.

1926   Rock, who graduated from Harvard Medical School, opens an infertility clinic at the Free Hospital for Women in Brookline, Massachusetts.

1928   Scientists identify the ovarian hormone progesterone, which plays a key role in pregnancy. A year later the sex hormone estrogen is also identified.

1932   Aldous Huxley's futurist novel *Brave New World* is published. It depicts a bleak society populated by test tube babies and shapes public perceptions of ART.

1934   Harvard scientist Gregory Pincus conducts IVF experiments involving rabbits that suggest similar fertilization is possible in humans. Pincus is denounced for his work, and Harvard denies him tenure.

1937   An unsigned editorial ("Conception in a Watch Glass") in the *New England Journal of Medicine*, written by John Rock, praises the possibilities of IVF: "What a boon for the barren woman with closed tubes to attempt such fertilization in humans." He hires Pincus's former technician Miriam Menkin as a research assistant.

1938   Hans Spemann theorizes that animals could be cloned by fusing an embryo with an egg cell; frozen sperm works for first time.

1943   Doris Del-Zio, who will become part of the first American IVF attempt, is born.

1944   In the six years since beginning their experiments, John Rock and Miriam Menkin collected some 800 ova and tried unsuccessfully to fertilize 138 of them. Between February and April, however, Menkin allows the egg and sperm to remain in contact for a longer period and succeeds in fertilizing four ova. This marks the first successful IVF of human eggs. Rock and Menkin do not attempt to implant the fertilized eggs in a woman. The published account of the research generates great interest.

The first meeting of the American Society for the Study of Human Sterility was held; later it was renamed the American society of Reproductive Medicine (ASRM).

1945   The *British Medical Journal* publishes early reports of AI using donor sperm, raising concerns in both the press and in Parliament.

1949   Pope Pius XII condemns any fertilization of human eggs outside the body, declaring that those who do so "take the Lord's work into their own hands." Despite Catholic Church resistance, the number of infertility clinics in the United States soars in the postwar era.

1951   Physician Landrum Shettles duplicates the Rock-Menkin experiments at Columbia-Presbyterian Hospital in New York City.

1954   A step back for science when an Illinois court rules that babies conceived through AI by donor are legally illegitimate. Most other states reject this. By 1960 some 50,000 babies have been born from a donor AI.

First successful pregnancy using frozen sperm.

1959   MC Change provides indisputable evidence of IVF obtained from the fertilization of rabbit ova. This opens the door to assisted procreation.

1961   Italian scientist Daniele Petrucci claims to have successfully fertilized 40 eggs and grown one embryo in the laboratory for 29 days (by which point it had developed a heartbeat) before destroying it. Although other scientists are skeptical of Petrucci's claim, the Vatican takes him at his word and denounces the experiment as sacrilegious.

Palmer from France describes the first retrieval of oocytes by laparoscopy.

1962   Shettles will later claim that in this year he transplanted a fertilized egg into a woman's uterus, resulting in a pregnancy. If true, this would be a landmark event, but Shettles's claim is never substantiated.

1965   British scientist Robert Edwards, who has been conducting unsuccessful fertilization experiments for many years, arrives in America and meets doctors Howard and Georgeanna Jones, who are working at Baltimore's Johns Hopkins University. The Joneses agree to help Edwards and to fertilize human eggs in vitro.

1966   The National Institutes of Health (NIH) sets out standards for all research performed by its grantees. In addition, the Department of Health, Education, and Welfare issues an order governing all clinical research conducted with federal grants. As a condition for receiving government money, universities with medical schools such as Columbia are required to sign letters pledging to abide by the guidelines in all research, not just the work directly funded by the government.

1967   First domestic household-based family planning survey of reproductive-aged women (Atlanta, Georgia).

1968   A computerized patient records system for family planning evaluation is developed.

Edwards, who has decided to try and implant fertilized eggs back into previously infertile women, meets Patrick Steptoe at a London gathering of the Royal Society of Medicine. Steptoe is a gynecologist in Oldham, England, who has developed a new technique of abdominal surgery called laparoscopy that may allow the retrieval of a mature human egg. Edwards and Steptoe agree to join forces to fertilize human eggs in vitro.

Pope Paul VI issues a papal encyclical called Humanae Vitae ("Of Human Life") that forbids Catholics from using contraceptives like the pill for birth control. Although IVF is not mentioned, the logic of Humanae Vitae, which requires the linkage of intercourse and procreation, seems to forbid external fertilization as well.

Doris and John Del-Zio marry. Doris, who is not 25 years old and has a daughter from a prior marriage, suffers a ruptured ovarian cyst and is subsequently unable to get pregnant. Later tests will reveal that her fallopian tubes are blocked.

1969   The first successful IVF of an immature human egg by Robert Edwards and Patrick Steptoe.

A Harris poll shows that most Americans believe techniques like IVF are against God's will. Edwards and Steptoe publish the result of their successful IVF experiments in the journal *Nature*. They have not yet attempted the implantation of fertilized eggs back into a woman.

First abortion surveillance report is published.

1970   An article appears in *Look* magazine called "Motherhood—Who Needs It?" The article opines that it doesn't make sense any more to pretend that women need babies when what they really need is themselves.

The next year, however, the magazine runs a cover feature entitled "The Test Tube Baby Is Coming" that trumpets Shettles's achievements in the field and makes him famous.

Doris Del Zio undergoes two operations to try and repair her fallopian tubes. In October she becomes pregnant, but Doris suffers a miscarriage at Christmas.

1971   Doris Del-Zio has yet another operation and then tries AI, which doesn't work.

Edwards and Steptoe's proposal for government funding is turned down by Great Britain's Medical Research Council. Meanwhile, in the United States the Human Embryo Research Panel is formed and charged with advising NIH whether to fund experiments involving human fetal tissue. After heated debate, the panel recommends such funding, but its report is ignored.

At a Washington conference on biomedical ethics attended by Edwards and Nobel laureate James Watson, who with Francis Crick had uncovered the double helix structure of DNA, concludes that IVF research will necessitate infanticide. Edwards, who responds with a forceful defense of his work, is rewarded with a standing ovation.

1972   The American Medical Association urges a moratorium on IVF research involving humans, while the American Fertility Society (headed by Georgeanna Jones) urges further work in the field; a U.S. scientist fertilizes an egg in vitro.

1973   The Supreme Court issues its watershed decision in *Roe v. Wade*, legalizing abortion. Antiabortion activists have also expressed opposition to IVF because experiments typically involve the destruction of embryos.

The *Washington Post* reports on a brain development experiment in which a scientist decapitates aborted fetuses, sparking a furor and increasing government skittishness about funding IVF research.

Early in the morning, Doris Del-Zio, who has been on fertility drugs for over half a year, has follicular fluid containing eggs surgically removed from her ovaries by Dr. William Sweeney. Her husband, John, then takes the two test tubes containing the eggs to Columbia-Presbyterian Hospital. Shettles meets John Del-Zio in the lobby and sends him to the bathroom to collect a sperm sample. Shettles then takes the tubes to a research laboratory, mixes the fluid and sperm together, and leaves it in an incubator. His plan is to allow the mixture to fertilize for four days and then implant it in Doris's uterus. Later that day a colleague in whom Shettles has confided alerts her superior about the experiment.

Early in the morning, news of Shettles's work reaches department chairman Raymond Vande Wiele, who orders the Del-Zio test tube brought to him. Vande Wiele, who believes the experiment will jeopardize Columbia's federal grants and has grown weary of Shettles's continued refusals to follow hospital procedure, summons Shettles to a meeting. Around 2 p.m. Vande Wiele confronts Shettles with the test tube, which has been at room temperature for several hours and whose contents can no longer be used. John Del-Zio learns about Columbia's actions from Sweeney, and later that evening, Doris, still recovering from her surgery, hears from Shettles what has happened. Her attempt to have another child has failed again. Under pressure from hospital administrators, Shettles resigns from Columbia-Presbyterian.

The Monash research team in Australia reports the first IVF pregnancy, which unfortunately results in early miscarriage.

1974   The publication of an Intrauterine Device Morbidity and Mortality study.

In the month her child would have been born, Doris Del-Zio claims that she woke up from a faint in a Florida department store to find her arms full of baby clothes. Later that summer the Del-Zios file suit against Vande Wiele and Columbia-Presbyterian for intentional infliction of emotional distress, seeking $1.5 million in damages.

British gynecology professor Douglas Bevis claims to have shepherded three test tube babies through to successful birth, but the children cannot be found and Bevis's claim is never substantiated.

The National Infertility Association, also known as RESOLVE, is established.

1975   The first international contraceptive prevalence survey is published.

Robert Edwards and Patrick Steptoe have the first successful IVF pregnancy, but it is an ectopic pregnancy, which implants in the fallopian tubes instead of the uterus, and the baby is lost. The medical team decides to stop giving their patients fertility drugs and instead focus on surgical retrieval of a single egg that will then be fertilized.

The U.S. government decides that federal grants can only be used for fetal research if they are first approved by a National Ethics Advisory Board. But this board will not be created until January 1978, effectively freezing IVF research in the United States throughout the mid-1970s.

The debate on the status of the human embryo ends government research on human embryos from IVF procedures.

1976   Twenty-nine-year-old former cheese factory worker Lesley Brown and her husband John meet with Steptoe. Lesley has blocked fallopian tubes, and Steptoe proposes IVF as a solution. The Browns agree.

Attorney Noel Keane arranges the first surrogate motherhood contract.

1977   The first IVF pregnancy is achieved; however, it is an unsuccessful pregnancy.

Howard and Georgeanna Jones retire after a combined 85 years of teaching at Johns Hopkins and are lured to the Eastern Virginia Medical School in Norfolk by an old friend.

Steptoe surgically removes an egg from Lesley Brown's ovaries. Two days later the fertilized egg developed into an eight-cell embryo, which he then implants into Lesley's uterus.

Edwards and Steptoe discover that Lesley is pregnant; the egg that was fertilized in vitro has become the very first one to grow in utero.

1978   After discovering that theirs will be the world's first test tube baby and becoming subjects of a media feeding frenzy, the Browns attempt to diminish the chaos by selling rights to the story to a British tabloid for half a million dollars.

Louise Brown, the first IVF or "test tube" baby is born in England.

The Collaborative Review of Sterilization (CREST) begins; the Division of Reproductive Health (DRH) investigates the safety and efficacy of sterilization procedures in the United States.

The earliest record of harvesting a dead man's sperm to use for conception is documented.

1979   The first tracking of the growth of follicles by ultrasound.

1980   The first IVF birth in Australia; first international meeting on IVF is held in Germany.

1981   A global survey of sterilization deaths is published; the Family Planning Evaluation Division was renamed the Division of Reproductive Health.

Elizabeth Jordan Carr, the first American baby to be conceived by IVF, is born in Norfolk, Virginia.

The introduction of Clomiphene citrate (Clomid) and hMG to induce the development of multiple eggs.

1982   The first births of French, Swedish, and Austrian IVF babies; Division of Reproductive Health investigates the relationship between cancer and the use of oral contraceptives; the World Health Organization (WHO) designates the Division of Reproductive Health as a Collaborating Center in Perinatal Mortality and in Family Planning.

Family Planning Methods and Practice: Africa is published; first report on the Canadian IVF baby; world's first IVF triplets born.

1984   First baby, Zoe Leyland, born from a frozen embryo. First baby born using a donated egg. Surveillance of infant mortality; also, the first surrogacy embryo transfer baby born in California.

1985   First reported birth after replacement of a hatching blastocyst cryopreserved at the expanded blastocyst stage; first IVF twins born from frozen embryos in Australia.

1986   The Cancer and Steroid Hormones Study concludes that the birth control pill does not cause cancer and decreases the risk for certain kinds of cancer; surveillance of maternal mortality is initiated; initiated a national strategy to examine and prevent prematurity in the United States; Maternal and Child Health Epidemiology bureau is established.

Gamete intrafallopian transfer (GIFT) and zygote intrafallopian transfer (ZIFT) technologies are first successfully used.

First mention of the term "embryo adoption" in the legal literature.

1987   Pregnancy Risk Assessment Monitoring System is developed.

The embryo transfer procedure is patented, starting a trend among fertility specialists of patenting the processes and products of human tissue manipulation.

**1988–
1989**   Australia's first IVF surrogate birth.
The surrogacy case of Baby M comes before the courts when surrogate mother Mary Beth Whitehead refuses to surrender custody of the child she carried for another couple. The New Jersey court awards the baby's genetic father and his wife permanent custody but allows Whitehead visitation rights.

First report on the use of laser techniques in ART for application in gametes and embryos.

1990   Infant health initiative preterm delivery research program is established; first report of assisted hatching in human embryos.

1991   Project CARES (Comprehensive AIDS and Reproductive Health Education Study) is implemented.

Arlette Schweitzer, 42, becomes mother of her grandchild by serving as a gestational surrogate for her daughter.

1992   First successful pregnancy using intracytoplasmic sperm injection (ICSI);

Fertility Clinic Success Rates and Certification Act of 1992 passed.

SIDS case control studies launched.

1993   The National Institutes of Health Revitalization Act sponsors research in IVF and related techniques.

1994   Book *From Data to Action: CDC's Public Health Surveillance for Women, Infants and Children* is published.

The first live birth of IVM following transvaginal ultrasound-guided oocyte collection. In vitro maturation and the fertilization and developmental competence of oocytes recovered from untreated polycystic ovarian patients.

1995   Teenage Pregnancy Prevention initiative established. First United States–based reproductive health survey of immigrant population is conducted.

The first report of aneuploidy testing (an abnormal number of chromosomes in a cell).

1996   Twins born of dead man's sperm win rights when mother Lauren Woodward sues and wins Social Security for her twin daughters.

1997   First successful birth using frozen eggs.

CDC releases the first annual report of pregnancy success rates for fertility clinics in the United States.

World's first cytoplasmic transfer birth at Saint Barnabas Medical Center in New Jersey. Cytoplasm from a donor egg is injected into the egg of a woman considered unable to sustain a pregnancy but who would like to have a genetic connection to a child. Since cytoplasm has mitochondrial DNA, the resulting embryo carries the genetic material from the sperm and both women (the egg donor and the infertile woman). Considered the first inroad into germline genetic manipulation.

Birth of McCaughey septuplets.

1998   Reproductive Health for Refugees initiative; Baby Hannah becomes the first baby born via donated embryos through the Snowflakes Frozen Embryo Adoption Program.

The first instance of a woman using sperm collected after a man's death to get pregnant.

1999   Launch of the CDC's Division of Reproductive Health website; first unaffected pregnancy using PGD for sickle cell anemia.

2000   Children's Health Act of 2000, which established Safe Motherhood; first birth using cryopreserved oocytes and frozen sperm.

Linda and Jack Nash decide to have a "savior child," who can donate bone marrow to older daughter Molly, who has Fanconi anemia, a disease that leads to bone marrow failure. Doctors use PGD to find the right donor match from the fertilized embryos. The second child donates cells from her umbilical cord.

2001   First National Summit on Safe Motherhood is held; scientists say they can create designer sperm.

2002   The Women's CARE study concludes that oral contraceptive use is not associated with a significantly increased risk of breast cancer; first live birth following blastocyst biopsy and PGD analysis.

2003   Sixty-five-year-old becomes the oldest known woman in the world to give birth using donated eggs from her niece and donated sperm from her niece's husband.

Online Interactive Atlas of Reproductive Health is launched. Division of Reproductive Health begins working in Afghanistan to reduce maternal and neonatal morbidity and mortality. Initiated a national strategy to examine and prevent prematurity in the United States.

A San Diego woman sues her physician for being denied AI because she is a lesbian.

2004   First preimplantation HLA matching for stem cell transplantation to an affected sibling; first report of fertility preservation for cancer patients using in vitro maturation and oocyte vitrification; first report on oocyte cryopreservation to save fertility in cancer patients; the first reported live birth following preimplantation genetic diagnosis for retinoblastoma.

2005   Science-based approaches are promoted to prevent teen pregnancy, HIV, and STDs.

2007   Expert panel consultation on youth development as a strategy to promote adolescent reproductive health; introduction of the concept of Milt Treatment Strategy for IVF.

2008   A CDC-wide working group is convened to examine the issue of infertility in the United States.

2009   CDC is an outreach partner participating in development of context.

2010   A National Public Health Action Plan for the Detection, Prevention, and Management of Infertility is released.

Division of Reproductive Health in collaboration with the Division of Adolescent and School Health and university partners publishes a special supplement on the importance of Positive Youth Development for Adolescent Reproductive Health Outcomes.

A National Public Health Action Plan for the Detection, Prevention, and Management of Infertility is released.

2011   Division of Reproductive Health and U.S. Agency for International Development completed a 37-year agreement to provide technical and scientific assistance for global reproductive health.

2012   The newly established Embryo Donation Services Center (EDSC) provides consultation services at no charge to embryo donors and adopters.

PRAMS (Pregnancy Risk Assessment Monitoring System) expands to 41 sites representing 78 percent of all U.S. live births.

CDC's *Vital Signs* releases first featured report on preventing teen pregnancy.

2014   CDC and the U.S. Office of Population Affairs jointly release *Providing Quality Family Planning Services* recommendations.

2015   Division of Reproductive Health publishes the first national report of gestational weight gain surveillance in pregnant women, noting the percent meeting gestational weight gain recommendations.

2016   Division of Reproductive Health responds to Zika.

Sources for Further Information

Books

Dunkel-Schetter C and Annette L. Stanton eds. 1991. "Psychological Adjustment to Infertility," in *Infertility: Perspectives from Stress and Coping Research*. The Springer Series on Stress and Coping. Boston: Springer.

Greely, Henry T. 2016. *The End of Sex and the Future of Human Reproduction*. Cambridge: Harvard University Press.

Inhorn, Marcia C. 2015. *Cosmopolitan Conceptions: IVF Sojourns in Global Dubai*. Durham: Duke University Press.

Kasky, Jeffrey A. and Marla Neufeld. 2016. *ABA Guide to Assisted Reproduction: Techniques, Legal Issues, and Pathways to Success*. Chicago: American Bar Association.

Macklon, Nick S., Human M. Fatermi, Robert J. Norman, and Pasquale Patrizio eds. 2015. *Case Studies in Assisted Reproduction: Common and Uncommon Presentations*. Cambridge: Cambridge University Press.

McHaffie, Hazel. 2014. *Saving Sebastian*. Edinburgh: Luath Press Ltd.

Picoult, Jodi. 2004. *My Sister's Keeper*. New York: Washington Square Press.

Roberts, Dorothy. 1997. *Killing the Black Body: Race, Reproduction and the Meaning of Liberty*. New York: Pantheon.

Rochman, Bonnie. 2017. *The Gene Machine: How Genetic Technologies Are Changing the Way We Have Kids—and the Kids We Have*. New York: Scientific American/Farrar, Straus and Giroux.

Shaw, Elizabeth and Chef Sara Haas. 2017. *Fertility Foods Cookbook: 100+ Recipes to Nourish Your Body*. Long Island City, NY: Hatherleigh Press.

Spar, Debora L. 2006. *The Baby Business: How Money, Science, and Politics Drive the Commerce of Conception.* Boston: Harvard Business School Press.

Speier, Amy. 2016. *Fertility Holidays: IVF Tourism and the Reproduction of Whiteness.* New York: NYU Press.

Sterngass, Jon. 2011. *Reproductive Technology.* Salt Lake City: Benchmark Books.

Taylor-Sands, Michelle. 2013. *Saviour Siblings: A Relational Approach to the Welfare of the Child in Selective Reproduction.* New York: Routledge.

Zoll, Miriam. 2013. *Cracked Open: Liberty, Fertility, and the Pursuit of High-Tech Babies.* Northampton: Interlink Publishing Group.

ORGANIZATIONS

American Academy of Adoption Attorneys
http://www.adoptionattorneys.org/aaaa/home
An organization of attorneys who must be licensed for at least five years and have acted as lead counsel in at least 50 adoption proceedings, including 10 interstate (ICPC) compact placements for children in the two years prior to being invited to join the Academy.

American Academy of Assisted Reproductive Technology Attorneys
http://www.aaarta.org/aaarta/home
An organization of attorneys who have completed at least 50 diverse ARTs matters prior to being invited to join AAARTA. The matters must include such legal services as obtaining parentage or birth orders, drafting and negotiating surrogacy, egg donor and sperm donor contracts, and drafting or reviewing embryo donation contracts.

American College of Medical Genetics (ACMG)
https://www.acmg.net/
An organization composed of biochemical, clinical, cytogenetic, medical, and molecular geneticists; genetic counselors; and other healthcare professionals.

American Fertility Association
http://www.path2parenthood.org/
An inclusive organization committed to helping people create their families by providing leading-edge outreach programs and timely educational information. The scope of work encompasses reproductive health, infertility prevention and treatment, and family-building options including adoption and third-party solutions.

American Pregnancy Association
www.americanpregnancy.org
A national health organization committed to promoting reproductive and pregnancy wellness through education, support, advocacy, and community awareness.

American Society for Reproductive Medicine
www.asrm.org
The nationally and internationally recognized leader for multidisciplinary information, education, advocacy, and standards in the field of reproductive medicine; it is a nonprofit whose members demonstrate the high ethical principles of the medical profession and an interest in infertility, reproductive medicine, and biology.

Baby Quest Foundation
http://babyquestfoundation.org/
Baby Quest Foundation provides financial assistance through fertility grants to those who cannot afford the high costs of procedures such as IVF (in vitro fertilization), gestational surrogacy, egg and sperm donation, egg freezing, artificial insemination, and embryo donation.

Cade Foundation
http://www.cadefoundation.org/
An organization started in 2005 to provide information, support, and financial assistance to help needy families overcome infertility. It provides education-focused programs to share information about different pathways to parenthood throughout the nation. It also provides grants to help families with the costs of adoption and fertility treatment.

Center for Bioethics and Culture
http://www.cbc-network.org/
This organization addresses bioethical issues that most profoundly affect our humanity, especially issues that arise in the lives of the most vulnerable among us; the network works through a variety of media platforms—documentary film, writing, speaking, interviews, social media, and more—to educate and inform members of the public, thought leaders, lawmakers, and others on ethical issues in healthcare, biomedical research, and biotechnological advancement.

Center for Genetics and Society
http://www.geneticsandsociety.org
A nonprofit social justice organization that works to ensure an equitable future where human genetic and reproductive technologies benefit the common good.

Creating a Family
www.creatingafamily.org
The national adoption and infertility education organization whose mission is to strengthen families through unbiased education and support for infertility patients, adoptive parents, and allied professionals.

European Society of Human Reproduction and Embryology
https://www.eshre.eu/Home/About-us.aspx
An organization to promote interest in, and understanding of, reproductive biology and medicine through facilitating research and subsequent dissemination of research findings in human reproduction and embryology to the public, scientists,

clinicians, and patient associations; it also works to collaborate with politicians and policy makers throughout Europe.

Fertile Action
http://www.fertileaction.org/
A cancer charity working to ensure fertile women touched by the disease can become mothers. Specifically, it educates, advocates, supports, and provides financial aid.

Fertility for Colored Girls
www.fertilityforcoloredgirls.org
An organization that seeks to provide education, awareness, support, and encouragement to African American women/couples and other women of color experiencing infertility and seeking to build the families of their dreams; it also seeks to empower African American women to take charge of their fertility and reproductive health.

Fertility within Reach
http://www.fertilitywithinreach.org/
Through education and coaching, Fertility within Reach aims to empower infertile individuals to advocate to build their family. Information is intended to support the communication process with physicians, insurance companies, employers, and legislators in collaborative efforts to access infertility treatment for yourself and the infertility community.

Genetics & IVF Institute
https://www.givf.com/
The Genetics & IVF Institute is a fully integrated, comprehensive fertility organization and center in Fairfax, Virginia (Washington, D.C., metropolitan area). Since 1984, it has been an innovator in infertility treatment and genetics care and has helped thousands of patients worldwide realize their dreams of starting a family.

The Hastings Center
http://www.thehastingscenter.org
The world's first bioethics research institute, it is a nonpartisan, nonprofit organization of research scholars from multiple disciplines, including philosophy, law, political science, and education; it produces books, articles, and other publications on ethical questions in medicine, science, and technology that help inform policy, practice, and public understanding.

The International Committee Monitoring Assisted Reproductive Technologies
www.icmartivf.org
An independent, international nonprofit organization that has taken a leading role in the development, collection, and dissemination of worldwide data on assisted reproductive technology; it provides information on availability, effectiveness, and safety to health professionals, health authorities, and to the public.

International Council on Infertility Information Dissemination (INCIID)
http://www.inciid.org/

A nonprofit organization that helps individuals and couples explore their family-building options. It provides current information and immediate support regarding the diagnosis, treatment, and prevention of infertility and pregnancy loss and offers guidance to those considering adoption or childfree lifestyles.

The International Society for Mild Approaches in Assisted Reproduction
http://ismaar.org/
An organization aimed at promoting education, training, and research into mild approaches in assisted reproduction and women's reproductive health in general.

Livestrong Fertility
https://www.livestrong.org/we-can-help/livestrong-fertility
An organization that provides information about the risks of infertility from cancer treatments and family-building options; it helps you understand how your fertility can be affected by cancer and cancer treatments and how to plan your family before, during, and after cancer.

Men Having Babies
http://www.menhavingbabies.org/
A nonprofit organization that was spun off in July 2012 from a program that ran at the NYC LGBT Center since 2005. It started as a peer support network for biological gay fathers and fathers-to-be, offering monthly workshops and an annual seminar. Over time, elaborate online resources were developed, the group's mailing expanded to about 2,000 couples and singles from around the world, and it teamed up with LGBT family associations to develop similar programs in Chicago, San Francisco, Los Angeles, Barcelona, Tel Aviv, and Brussels.

National Certification Commission for Acupuncture and Oriental Medicine (NCCAOM)
http://www.nccaom.org/
A nonprofit established in 1982, it is the only national organization that validates entry-level competency in the practice of acupuncture and Oriental medicine (AOM) through professional certification.

National Embryo Donation Center
https://www.embryodonation.org/about/
Since 2003, this is the country's leading comprehensive nonprofit embryo donation program. Their mission is to protect the lives and dignity of human embryos and do that by promoting, facilitating, and educating about embryo donation and adoption. This is the only clinic-based organization that works with families of all races, faiths, and ethnic backgrounds.

Religious Coalition for Reproductive Choice
www.Rcrc.org
An organization that coordinates an interfaith movement that brings the moral force of religion to protect and advance reproductive health, choice, rights, and justice through education, prophetic witness, pastoral presence, and advocacy.

Religious Institute
http://www.religiousinstitute.org

A multifaith organization dedicated to advocating for sexual, gender, and reproductive health, education, and justice in faith communities and society.

Reproductive Health Technologies Project
http://rhtp.org
Organization to advance the ability of every woman of any age to achieve full reproductive freedom with access to the safest, most effective, appropriate, and acceptable technologies for ensuring her own health and controlling her fertility; it seeks to build consensus in support of an education, research, and advocacy agenda for reproductive health and reproductive freedom.

RESOLVE
www.Resolve.org
The National Infertility Association, established in 1974 and dedicated to ensuring that all people challenged in their family-building journey reach resolution through being empowered by knowledge, supported by community, united by advocacy, and inspired to act.

Snowflakes Embryo Adoption Program
https://www.nightlight.org/snowflakes-embryo-adoption-donation/embryo-adoption/
A child-centered adoption agency that finds loving families for children and believes in the open adoption model when placing kids for adoption.

Society of Assisted Reproductive Technology
www.sart.org
The primary organization of professionals dedicated to the practice of assisted reproductive technologies in the United States.

Uprooted
http://weareuprooted.org/
An organization born from the idea that one can feel *uprooted* from one's self, one's community, one's vision for the future, and one's body when going through family-building struggles. Often, those struggling to grow their families feel isolated from the Jewish community both socially and spiritually. Through programming, advocacy, and ritual creation, Uprooted educates American Jewish leaders in assisting families with fertility challenges and provides national communal support to those struggling to grow their families.

Urge
http://urge.org
An organization that engages young people in creating and leading the way to sexual and reproductive justice for all by providing training, field mobilization, and national leadership for a youth-driven agenda.

The Walking Egg
www.thewalkingegg.com
A nonprofit organization that strives to raise awareness about childlessness in resource-poor countries. It wants to make fertility care, including assisted reproductive technologies, available and accessible to a much larger proportion of the population.

ARTICLES

Abramowicz, Jacques S. 2017. "Ultrasound in Assisted Reproductive Technologies and the First Trimester: Is There a Risk?" *Clinical Obstetrics & Gynecology.*

Abrams, Papula. 2015. "The Bad Mother: Stigma, Abortion and Surrogacy." *Abortion and Art.*

Adams, Sarah. 2013. "Pre-Conception Detoxification." *High Tech Health Newsletter International.*

Adamson, G. David and Mary E. Abusief. 2016. "Fertility." *OBG Management.*

Ahmad, Eman Mjalli et al. 2016. "What to Expect from an In Vitro Fertilization/ Preimplantation Genetic Diagnosis and Gender Selection Program for Family Balancing?" *IVF Lite.*

Alasmari, Nouf M. et al. 2016. "The Effect on Pregnancy and Multiples of Transferring 1-3 Embryos in Women at Least 40 Years Old." *Journal of Assisted Reproduction and Genetics.*

Allen, Brian D. et al. 2014. "On the Cost and Prevention of Iatrogenic Multiple Pregnancies. *Reproductive BioMedicine Online.*

Allen, Reniqua. 2016. "Is Egg Freezing Only for White Women?" *New York Times.*

Allen, Samantha. 2014. "The Artificial Womb Will Change Feminism Forever." *Daily Beast.*

Alter, Charlotte. 2015. "Buying Time." *TIME.* http://time.com/3960528/the-truth -about-freezing-your-eggs/.

American Pregnancy Association. 2017. "Female Infertility." http:// americanpregnancy.org/infertility/female-infertility.

"An arm and Leg for a Fertilised Egg." 2016. *The Economist.* https://www .economist.com/news/briefing/21705676-doctors-have-spent-decades-trying -make-ivf-more-effective-now-they-trying -to-make-it.

Appold, Karen. 2014. "Preimplantation Genetic Diagnosis: How Should Labs Grapple with Ethics?" *Clinical Laboratory News.*

Arousell, Jonna and Aje Carlborn. 2016. "Culture and Religious Beliefs in Relation to Reproductive Health." *Best Practice & Research Clinical Obstetrics and Gynaecology.*

Arya, Shafali Talisa and Bridget Dibb. 2016. "The Experience of Infertility Treatment: The Male Perspective." *Human Fertility.*

Asch, Adrienne and Rebecca Marmor. 2009. "Hastings Center Bioethics Briefings for Journalists, Policymakers, and Educators: Assisted Reproduction." Hastings Center.

Asgarini, Najmeh et al. 2016. "Investigation of Personality Traits between Infertile Women Submitted to Assisted Reproductive Technology or Surrogacy." *International Journal of Fertility and Sterility.*

Bailey, Anna. 2016. "Coping and Resilience among Women Undergoing Assisted Reproductive Therapies." Dissertation for Canterbury Christ Church University.

Ball, Philip. 2016. "Immaculate Conceptions." *New Statesman.*

Baron, Keren Tuvia et al. 2012. "Emergent Complications of Assisted Reproduction: Expecting the Unexpected." *Radiology.*

Barton, Sara E. et al. 2012. "Population-Based Study of Attitudes Toward Posthumous Reproduction. *Fertility and Sterility.*

Bay, Bjorn et al. 2013. "Assisted Reproduction and Child Neurodevelopmental Outcomes: A Systematic Review." *National Agricultural Library.*

Ben-Aviv, Michelle. 2016. "Why Infertility Is a Jewish Issue-and What We Can Do About It." *Washington Jewish Week.*

Bendeck, Odette Marie. 2014. "The Progeny of Florida's Reproductive Technology Statutes." *Florida Bar Journal.*

Benston, Shawna. 2016. "CRISPR, a Crossroads in Genetic Intervention: Pitting the Right to Health against the Right to Disability." *Laws.*

Bissonnette, Francois et al. 2011. "Working to Eliminate Multiple Pregnancies: a Success Story in Quebec." *Reproductive BioMedicine Online.*

Bjelica, Artur and Svetlana Nikolic. 2015. "Development and Achievements of Assisted Reproductive Technology." *Med Pregl.*

Black, Sheila. 2016. "Passing My Disability on to My Children." *New York Times.*

Blake, Lucy et al. 2016. "Gay Father Surrogacy Families: Relationships with Surrogates and Egg Donors and Parental Disclosure of Children's Origins." *Fertility and Sterility.*

Boggs, Belle, 2016. "The Price of Infertility." *The Cut.*

Boggs, Belle. 2016. "What No One Tells Couples Trying to Conceive." *The Cut.*

Boodman, Sandra G. 2016. "Do Women Who Donate Their Eggs Run a Health Risk?" *Washington Post.*

Booth, Molly E. 2015. "Donating Life: A Survey of the Ethical Consequences of Genetic Child Production by In Vitro Fertilization in Parental versus Donor Reproductive Material." *Rutgers Journal of Bioethics.*

Boulet, Sheree L. et al. 2016. "Assisted Reproductive Technology and Birth Defects among Liveborn Infants in Florida, Massachusetts, and Michigan, 2000–2010." *JAMA Pediatrics.*

Brody, Jane E. 2016. "Some I.V.F. Experts Discourage Multiple Births." *New York Times.*

Brown, Hannah. 2016. "How Old Is Too Old for a Safe Pregnancy?" *The Conversation.*

Brown, Herbert N. and Martin J. Kelly. 1976. "Stages of Bone Marrow Transplantation: A Psychiatric Perspective." *Psychosomatic Medicine.*

Busch, Morten. 2017. "Women Can Write Themselves Out of a Fertility Crisis." *Novo Nordisk Fonden.*

Campbell, Alexia Fernandez. 2015. "Five Myths about Women of Color, Infertility, and IVF Debunked." *Atlantic.*

Carbone, June and Jody Lynee Madeira. 2016. "Buyers in the Baby Market: Toward a Transparent Consumerism." *Washington Law Review.*

Cassidy, Tony and Marian McLaughlin. 2016. "Distress and Coping with In Vitro Fertilisation (IVF): The Role of Self-Compassion, Parenthood Motivation and Attachment." *Journal of Psychology and Clinical Psychiatry.*

Cederblad, M. et al. 1996. "Children: Intelligence and Behaviour in Children Born After In-Vitro Fertilization Treatment."*Human Reproduction.*

Chapman, Jennifer E. and Mark Zhang. 2013. "Davis v. Davis (1992)." *The Embryo Project Encyclopedia.*

Charo, R. Alta. 2016. "The Legal and Regulatory Context for Human Gene Editing." *Issues in Science and Technology.*

Chiles, Kelly A. and Peter N. Schlegel. 2016. "Cost-Effectiveness of Varicocele Surgery in the Era of Assisted Reproductive Technology." *Asian Journal of Andrology.*

Clark, Shannon M. 2016. "I'm a High-Risk Pregnancy Expert. So Why Didn't I Worry About My Own Fertility?" *Washington Post.*

Colban, Jill. 2016. "Out of the Goodness of My Heart, I Give You This Child." *Seton Hall Law Paper.*

Conley, Mikaela. 2011. "Israel Court Allows Family to Harvest Dead Daughter's Eggs." *ABC News.*

Conrad, Hannah Lynn. 2012. "Guiding Patients through Infertility Given the Current Ethical Views on ART from Catholic, Christian-Protestant, Jewish and Islamic Faith Traditions." Dissertation for the University of Toledo.

Cook, Rebecca J. and Bernard M. Dickens. 2014. "Reducing Stigma in Reproductive Health." *International Journal of Gynecology and Obstetrics.*

Corley-Newman, Antoinette. 2016. "The Relationship between Infertility, Infertility Treatment, Therapeutic Interventions, and Post-Traumatic Stress Disorder." *Dissertation for Walden University.*

Cortez, Nathan. 2008. "Patients without Borders: The Emerging Global Market for Patients and the Evolution of Modern Health Care." *Indiana Law Journal.*

Cromi, A. et al. 2016. "Risks of Peripartum Hysterectomy in Births after Assisted Reproductive Technology." *Fertility and Sterility.*

Cummings, Mike. 2015. "Q&A with Marcia Inhorn: IVF Sojourners in Dubai." *Yale News.*

Cutas, Daniela and Anna Smajdor. 2016. "I Am Your Mother and Your Father! In Vitro Derived Gametes and the Ethics of Solo Reproduction." *Health Care Analysis.*

De La Cruz, Donna. 2016. "Should Young Women Sell Their Eggs?" *New York Times.*

Deonandan, Raywat. 2015. "Recent Trends in Reproductive Tourism and International Surrogacy: Ethical Considerations and Challenges for Policy." *Risk Management and Healthcare Policy.*

Dimond, Rebecca. 2015. "Social and Ethical Issues in Mitochondrial Donation." *British Medical Bulletin.*

Domar, Alice D. 2017. "Psychological Stress and Infertility." *UpToDate.*

Drosdzol, Agnieszka. 2009. "Depression and Anxiety Among Polish Infertile Couples—an Evaluative Prevalence Study." *Journal of Psychosomatic Obstetrics & Gynecology.*

Dupree, James. 2016. "Insurance Coverage for Male Infertility Care in the United States." *Asian Journal of Andrology.*

Eisenberg, Amanda. 2016. "Flexibility Family-Friendly Benefits Gaining Momentum." *Employee Benefit News.*

Elliott, Peter et al. 2016. "Out-of-Pocket Costs for Men Undergoing Infertility Care and Associated Financial Strain." *Urology Practice.*

Environment and Reproductive Health Study Team. 2016. "Serum 25-Hydroxy-Vitamin D Concentrations and Treatment Outcomes of Women Undergoing Assisted Reproduction." *American Journal of Clinical Nutrition.*

ESHRE. 2015. "Largest Study of Babies Born After Infertility Treatment Shows Significant Improvements in Health Over Past 20 Years." *European Society of Human Reproduction and Embryology.*

Estes, Jaclyn. 2015. "The Ethics of Pre-Implantation Genetic Testing." *Rutgers Journal of Bioethics.*

Fatemeh, Jafarzadeh Kenarsari. 2015. "Exploration of Infertile Couples' Support Requirements: A Qualitative Study." *International Journal of Fertility and Sterility.*

Fatima, Misbahul. 2015. "Minor Donations: Using Children as a Means to an End." *Seton Hall E Repository.*

Feichtinger, Michael and Kenny A. Rodriguez-Wallberg. 2016. "Fertility Preservation in Women with Cervical, Endometrial or Ovarian Cancers." *Gynecologic Oncology Research and Practice.*

Figueira, Rita C. S. et al. 2012. "Preimplantation Diagnosis for B-Thalassemia Combined with HLA Matching: First Savior Sibling Is Born after Embryo Selection in Brazil." *Journal of Assisted Reproduction and Genetics.*

Finkelstein, Alex et al. 2016. "Surrogacy Law and Policy in the U.S.: A National Conversation Informed by Global Lawmaking."*Columbia Law School.*

Fogleman, Sarah et al. 2016. "CRISPR/Cas9 and Mitochondrial Gene Replacement Therapy: Promising Techniques and Ethical Considerations." *American Journal of Stem Cells.*

Ford, Allison. 2017. "Designer Babies: Good Idea or Slippery Slope?" *The Atlantic.*

Fountain, Christine et al. 2015. "Association Between Assisted Reproductive Technology Conception and Autism in California, 1997–2007." *American Journal of Public Health.*

Fragouli, Elpida et al. 2015. "Altered Levels of Mitochondrial DNA Are Associated with Female Age, Aneuploidy and Provide an Independent Measure of Embryonic Implantation Potential." *PLOS Genetics.*

Friedersdorf, Conor. 2017. "Will Editing Your Baby's Genes Be Mandatory? *The Atlantic.*

Friedlander, Edwa et al. 2015. "Cognitive and Social-Communication Abilities among Young Children Conceived by Assisted Reproductive Technologies." *European Journal of Developmental Psychology.*

Galhardo, A. et al. 2016. "The Infertility Trap: How Defeat and Entrapment Affect Depressive Symptoms." *Human Reproduction.*

Gameiro, Sofia, et al. August 2016. "Birth outcomes and postpartum depression in women that conceived through assisted reproduction technologies." *Human Reproduction.*

Gameiro, S. August 2016. "Women's Adjustment Trajectories During IVF on Impact on Mental Health 11-17 Years Later." *Human Reproduction.*

Gitschier, Jane. 2014. "The Ethics of Our Inquiry: An Interview with Hank Greely." *PLOS Genetics.*

Gleicher, Norbert et al. 2014. "Regarding Euploid Single Embryo Transfer: The New IVF Paradigm." *Fertility and Sterility.*

Golombok, S. et al. 2006. "Non-Genetic and Non-Gestational Parenthood: Consequences for Parent–Child Relationships and the Psychological Well-Being of Mothers, Fathers and Children at Age 3." *Human Reproduction.*

Goswami, Shivani. 2016. "Womb for Rent: An Aid or a Sclotch?" *Valley International Journals.*

Grose, Jessica. 2015. "The Sherri Shepherd Surrogacy Case Is a Mess. Prepare for More Like It." *Slate.*

Haaf, Lisette Ten. 2016. "Future Persons and Legal Persons: The Problematic Representation of the Future Child in the Regulation of Reproduction." *Laws.*

Hajela, Supriya et al. "Stress and Infertility: A Review." *International Journal of Reproduction, Contraception and Obstetrical Gynecology.*

Hebert, Nicole. 2008. "Creating a Life to Save a Life: An Issue Inadequately Addressed by the Current Legal Framework under Which Minors Are Permitted to Donate Tissue and Organs." *Southern California Interdisciplinary Law Journal.*

Helft, Miguel. 2016. "End of the Biological Clock." *Forbes.*

Heng, B.C. et al. 2015. "Roles of Antiphospholipid Antibodies, Antithyroid Antibodies and Antisperm Antibodies in Female Reproductive Health." *Integrative Medicine International.*

Hjelmstedt, A. 2004. "Emotional Adaptation Following Successful In Vitro Fertilization." *Fertility and Sterility.*

Hofman, Darra L. 2009. "Mama's Baby, Daddy's Maybe: A State-by-State Survey of Surrogacy Law and Their Disparate Gender Impact." *William Mitchell Law Review.*

Humphries, Leigh A. et al. 2016. "Influence of Race and Ethnicity on In Vitro Fertilization Outcomes: Systematic Review." *American Journal of Obstetrics & Gynecology.*

Hvidtjorn, Dorte et al. 2009. "Cerebral Palsy, Autism Spectrum Disorders, and Developmental Delay in Children Born after Assisted Conception: A Systematic Review and Meta-Analysis." *JAMA's Archives of Pediatric Adolescent Medicine.*

Hyde, Jessica. 2017. "What Are the Recent Major Advances in Genetic Engineering?" *Quora.*

Inhorn, Marcia C. and Pasquale Patrizio. 2015. "Infertility around the Globe: New Thinking on Gender, Reproductive Technologies and Global Movements in the 21st Century." *Human Reproduction Update.*

Insogna, Iris G. and Elizabeth Ginsburg. 2016. "Transferring Embryos with Indeterminate PGD Results: The Ethical Implications." *Fertility Research and Practice.*

"Iodine Deficiency May Reduce Pregnancy Chances, NIH Study Suggests." 2018. *National Institutes of Health.*

Isasi, R. M. et al. 2016. "Supplementary Materials for Editing Policy to Fit the Genome?" *Science.*

Ishil, Tetsuya et al. 2013. "Ethical and Legal Issues Arising in Research on Inducing Human Germ Cells from Pluripotent Stem Cells." *Cell Stem Cell.*

"IVF Babies at Increased Risk for Developing Retinoblastoma." 2003. *Transplant News.*

Jafarzadeh-Kenarsari, F. et al. 2015. "Exploration of Infertile Couples' Support Requirements: A Qualitative Study." *International Journal of Fertility and Sterility.*

Jafarzadehpur, Ebrahim et al. 2013. "Ocular Manifestations in Infants Resulted from Assisted Reproductive Technology (ART)." *Journal of Family and Reproductive Health.*

James-Abra, S. et al. 2015. "Trans People's Experiences with Assisted Reproduction Services: A Qualitative Study." *Human Reproduction.*

Jindal, Sangita K. et al. 2016. "Guidelines for Handling Infectious Patients in the IVF Laboratory." *Reproductive BioMedicine Online.*

Jindal, Sangita K. et al. 2016. "Guidelines for Risk Reduction When Handling Gametes from Infectious Patients Seeking Assisted Reproductive Technologies." *Reproductive BioMedicine Online.*

Johnson, Katherine M. 2012. "Excluding Lesbian and Single Women? An Analysis of U.S. Fertility Clinic Websites." *Women's Studies International Forum.*

Jones, Ashby. 2015. "Putting a Price on a Human Egg; Lawsuit Claims Price Guidelines Used by Fertility Clinics Artificially Suppress the Amount Women Can Get for Their Eggs." *Wall Street Journal (online).*

Judd, Wes. 2015. "The Messy, Complicated Nature of Assisted Reproductive Technology." *Pacific Standard.*

Kamphuis, Esme I. 2014. "Are We Overusing IVF?" *British Medical Journal.*

Kang, Eunju et al. 2016. "Mitochondrial Replacement in Human Oocytes Carrying Pathogenic Mitochondrial DNA Mutations." *Nature.*

Karaca, Nilay et al. 2016. "Effect of IVF Failure on Quality of Life and Emotional Status in Infertile Couples." *European Journal of Obstetrics & Gynecology and Reproductive Biology.*

Karow, Julia. 2016. "Buoyed by National Screening Committee Recommendation, UK Providers Expect Demand for NIPT to Grow." *Genomeweb.*

Kawwass, Jennifer F. et al. 2015. "Safety of Assisted Reproductive Technology in the United States, 2000–2011." *JAMA.*

Kawwass, Jennifer F. et al. 2013. "Trends and Outcomes for Donor Oocyte Cycles in the United States, 2000–2010." *JAMA.*

Kindregan, Charles P. and Danielle White. 2013. "International Fertility Tourism: The Potential for Stateless Children in Cross-Border Commercial Surrogacy Arrangements." *Suffolk Transnational Law Review.*

Klitzman, Robert. 2016. "Deciding How Many Embryos to Transfer: Ongoing Challenges and Dilemmas." *Reproductive BioMedicine Online.*

Knaplund, Kristine S. 2014. "Assisted Reproductive Technology: The Legal Issues." *Probate & Property Magazine.*

Knapton, Sarah. 2016. "IVF Children Could Suffer Poorer Health, Warns Expert." *Daily Telegraph* (London, England).

Kristensen, David M. et al. 2018. "Ibuprofen Alters Human Testicular Physiology to Produce a State of Compensated Hypogonadism." *Proceedings of the National Academy of Sciences.*

Krupp, Deidre R. et al. 2017. "Exonic Mosaic Mutations Contribute Risk for Autism Spectrum Disorder." *American Journal of Human Genetics.*

Kumer, Dinka. 2016. "In Vitro Fertilization (IVF)." www.chabad.org.

Kushnir, Vitaly A. et al. 2017. "Systematic Review of Worldwide Trends in Assisted Reproductive Technology 2004–2013." *Reproductive Biology and Endocrinology.*

Lande, Yechezkel et al. 2011. "Couples Offered Free Assisted Reproductive Treatment Have a Very High Chance of Achieving a Live Birth Within 4 Years." *Fertility and Sterility.*

Lawson, Angela et al. 2016. "Blurring the Line Between Life and Death: A Review of the Psychological and Ethical Concerns Related to Posthumous-Assisted Reproduction." *European Journal of Contraception and Reproductive Health Care.*

Le Page, Michael. 2016. "Second CRISPR Human Embryo Study Shows There Is a Long Way to Go." www.newscientist.com.

Leary, Christine et al. 2015. "Human Embryos from Overweight and Obese Women Display Phenotypic and Metabolic Abnormalities." *Human Reproduction.*

Lee, Amy M. et al. 2016. "Elective Single Embryo Transfer—the Power of One." *Contraception and Reproductive Medicine.*

Legato, Marianne J. 2017. "Editing the Human Genome: Progress and Controversies." *Gender and the Genome.*

Leiser, Amy B. 2016. "Parentage Disputes in the Age of Mitochondrial Replacement Therapy." *Georgetown Law Journal.*

Levitt, Sarah. 2008. "Saviour Siblings: Genetic Screening and Policy." *The Meducator.*

Liss-Schultz, Nina. 2016. "The Despicable Way That Insurance Companies Screw over Lesbians." *Mother Jones.*

Litzky, Julia F. et al. 2017. "Placental Imprinting Variation Associated with Assisted Reproductive Technologies and Subfertility."*Epigenetics.*

Livingston, Gretchen. 2015a. "Is U.S. Fertility at an All-Time Low? It Depends." Pew Research Center.

Livingston, Gretchen. 2015b. "Twins, Triplets and More: More U.S. Births Are Multiples Than Ever Before." Pew Research Center.

Livingston, Shelby. 2016. "Fertility Treatment Costs Scare Off Employers." www.lbusinessinsurance.com.

Lones, Mark E. 2016. "A Christian Ethical Perspective on Surrogacy." *Bioethics in Faith and Practice.*

MacLeod, Kendra D. et al. 2003. "Pediatric Sibling Donors of Successful and Unsuccessful Hematopoietic Stem Cell Transplants (HSCT): A Qualitative Study of Their Psychosocial Experience." *Journal of Pediatric Psychology.*

Madeira, Jody Lynee and Barbara Andraka-Christou. 2016. "Paper Trails, Trailing Behind: Improving Informed Consent to IVF through Multimedia Applications." *Journal of Law and the Biosciences.*

Madrigal, Alexia C. 2014. "Making Babies." *Atlantic.*

Magelssen, Morten and Ole Jakob Filtvedt. 2015. "Assisted Reproduction, the Logic of Liberalization, and Five Christian Responses." *Ethics & Medicine.*

Mahmoud, Farouk. 2010. "Assisted Reproductive Technology (ART)—Ethics, Religion and the Law." *Sri Lanka Journal of Obstetrics and Gynaecology.*

Manninen, Bertha Alvarez. 2011. "Parental, Medical, and Sociological Responsibilities: Octomom as a Case Study in the Ethics of Fertility Treatments." *Journal of Clinical Research & Bioethics.*

Margalit, Yehezkel. 2016. "From Baby M to Baby M (anji): Regulating International Surrogacy Agreements." *Brooklyn Journal of Policy and Law.*

Martin, A. S. et al. 2016. "Risk of Preeclampsia in Pregnancies after Assisted Reproductive Technology and Ovarian Stimulation." *Maternal and Child Health Journal.*

Martin, Angela S. et al. 2016. "Trends in Severe Maternal Morbidity after Assisted Reproductive Technology in the United States, 2008–2012." *Obstetrics & Gynecology.*

Martins, Mariana V. et al. 2016. "Male Psychological Adaptation to Unsuccessful Medically Assisted Reproduction Treatments: A Systematic Review." *Marriage and Family Therapy.*

Matsumura, Kaiponanea T. 2017. "The End of Sex and the Future of Human Reproduction: Book Review." *Jurimetrics.*

May, Ashley. 2017. "What Your Religion Has to Say about How You Become a Parent." *USA Today.*

May, Joshua. 2015. "Emotional Reactions to Human Reproductive Cloning." *Reproductive Ethics.*

McQuillan, Julia et al. 2010. "Specifying the Effects of Religion on Medical Helpseeking: The Case of Infertility." *Social Science Medicine.*

Mesen, Tolga et al. 2015. "Optimal Timing for Elective Egg Freezing." *Fertility and Sterility.*

Miller, Valeria C. 2013. "Legal and Ethical Considerations on the Use of ART in the U.S. and Italy." www.digest.syr.edu.

Mills, Janelle, "Understanding the Position of the Savior Sibling." Thesis for Wake Forest University, December 2013, Winston Salem, NC.

Mirza, Salma et al. 2016. "Assisted Reproductive Technology (ART): A Review." *World Journal of Pharmacy and Pharmaceutical Sciences.*

Mohapatra, Seema. 2014. "Using Egg Freezing to Extend the Biological Clock: Fertility Insurance or False Hope?" *Harvard Law & Policy Review.*

Mortensen, Christina and Karin Stoeckenius. 2009. "Curing Discrimination: Many Doctors Refuse to Treat Lesbian Patients?" *Empire College Law Review.*

Motluk, Alison. 2015. "New Self-Incubated IVF Not Yet Cheaper." *Canadian Medical Association Journal.*

Nandy, Amrita. 2016. "Surrogacy Debate Fuels Stigma against Infertility." *Wire.*

Nargun, Geeta. 2015. "Scientific Evidence Shows the Need for a Fresh Approach to IVF." *Women's Health.*

"National Nutrient Database for Standard Reference." 2014. *National Agricultural Library.*

Naziri, Despina. 2015. "Unattainable Motherhood: A Psychodynamic Approach." www.in-fercit.gr.

Neimark, Jill. 2017. "Unexpected Risks Found in Replacing DNA to Prevent Inherited Disorders." *NPR Now.*

NeJaime, Douglas. 2015. "Griswold's Progeny: Assisted Reproduction, Procreative Liberty, and Sexual Orientation Equality." *Yale Law Journal Forum.*

"New Leukemia Findings from National Cancer Institute Discussed (Risk of Cancer in Children Conceived by Assisted Reproductive Technology. 2016. *Pediatrics Week.*

NHS Choices, ed. 2016. "IVF Not Proven to Cut Birth Defect Risk in Babies with Older Mothers." *States News Service.*

Nicolau, Yona et al. 2015. "Outcomes of Surrogate Pregnancies in California and Hospital Economics of Surrogate Maternity and Newborn Care." *World Journal of Obstetrics and Gynecology.*

Nonacs, Ruta. 2015. "Fertility Treatment May Increase the Risk of Postpartum Depression." *MGH Center for Women's Mental Health.*

Nwaru, Bright et al. 2016. "Assisted Reproductive Technology and Risk of Asthma and Allergy in the Offspring: Protocol for a Systematic Review and Meta-Analysis." *BMJ Open.*

O'Brien, Elizabeth. 2014. "10 Things Fertility Clinics Won't Tell You." *Marketwatch.*

O'Brien, Raymond. 2014. "The Momentum of Posthumous Conception: A Model Act." *Journal of Contemporary Health Law & Policy.*

Ollove, Michael. 2015. "Stateline: States Not Eager to Regulate Fertility Industry." *The Pew Charitable Trusts.*

Ombelet, W. and J. Van Robays. 2015. "Artificial Insemination History: Hurdles and Milestones." *Facts Views Vis Obgyn.*

"100-Year-Old Fertility Technique Reduces Need for IVF." 2017. *Science Daily.*

Opdahl, S. "Risk of Hypertensive Disorders in Pregnancies Following Assisted Reproductive Technology: A Cohort Study from the CONARTAS Group." *Human Reproduction.*

Ott, Kate M. 2009. "A Time to Be Born: A Faith-Based Guide to ARTs." www.religiousinstitute.org.

"Parenting and Personhood: Cross-Cultural Perspectives on Family-Life Expertise and Risk Management." 2016. *Canterbury Christ Church University.*

Patel, Ansha et al. 2016. "Prevalence and Predictors of Infertility-Specific Stress in Women Diagnosed with Primary Infertility: A Clinic-Based Study." *Journal of Human Reproductive Sciences.*

Perlyasamy, Anurekha Janaki et al. 2016. "Hepatitis B and C Virus in Assisted Reproductive Technology: A Review of Literature." *Women's Health & Gynecology.*

Persky, Anna Stolley. 2016. "Deep Freeze: Contentious Battles between Couples over Preserved Embryos Raise Legal and Ethical Dilemmas." *ABA Journal.*

Petok, William. 2015. "Infertility Counseling (or the Lack Thereof) of the Forgotten Male Partner." *Fertility and Sterility.*

Preidt, Robert. 2016. "Fewer Birth Defects for Older Moms Who Have Fertility Treatments." *Medline Plus.*

Provost, M. P. et al. 2016. "State Insurance Mandates and Multiple Birth Rates after In Vitro Fertilization." *Obstetrics and Gynecology.*

Radwan, M. et al. 2016. "Sperm DNA Damage—the Effect of Stress and Everyday Life Factors." *International Journal of Impotence Research.*

Rapaport, Lisa. 2016. "Reproductive Technology Linked to Birth Defects, Childhood Leukemia." *Reuters Health Medical News.*

Reardon, Sara. 2016. "Reports of 'Three Parent Babies' Multiply." *Nature News & Comment.*

Reimann, Maria. 2016. "I Was with My Wife the Entire Time. Polish Men's Narratives of IVF Treatment." *Reproductive BioMedicine and Society Online.*

"Reversing Male Infertility." 2018. *Ivanhoe*. https://www.ivanhoe.com/medical-breakthroughs/reversing-male-infertility/

Rexhaj, Emrush et al. "Mice Generated by In Vitro Fertilization Exhibit Vascular Dysfunction and Shortened Life Span." *The Journal of Clinical Investigation*.

Reznichenko, A. S. et al. 2015. "Mitochondrial Transfer: Ethical, Legal and Social Implications in Assisted Reproduction." *South Africa Journal of Bioethics and Law*.

Richard, Jeremie et al. 2016. "So Much of This Story Could Be Me: Men's Use of Support in Online Infertility Discussion Boards." *American Journal of Men's Health*.

Robey, Catherine. 2015. "Posthumous Semen Retrieval and Reproduction: An Ethical, Legal and Religious Analysis." Thesis for Wake Forest University.

Robson, Stephen J. et al. 2015. "Pregnancy and Childhood Health and Developmental Outcomes with the Use of Posthumous Human Sperm." *Human Reproduction*.

Roca-de Bes, Montserrat et al. 2011. "Comparative Study of the Psychosocial Risks Associated with Families with Multiple Births Resulting from Assisted Reproductive Technology (ART) and without ART." *Fertility and Sterility*.

Rodino, Iolanda S. et al. 2016. "Obesity and Psychological Wellbeing in Patients Undergoing Fertility Treatment." *Reproductive BioMedicine Online*.

Rosaria, Maria et al. 2016. "Anger in Women Treated with Assisted Reproductive Technology (ART): Effects on Mother and Newborn." *Journal of Maternal-Fetal and Neonatal Medicine*.

Rosenblum, Emma. 2014. "Later, Baby: Will Freezing Your Eggs Free Your Career?" *Bloomberg Business Week*.

Ross, Lori E. et al. 2011. "Risk for Postpartum Depression Associated with Assisted Reproductive Technologies and Multiple Births: A Systematic Review." *Human Reproduction Update*.

Rubin, Rita. 2016. "Bill to Cover Assisted Reproductive Technology for Some Veterans." *Journal of the American Medical Association*.

Russo, Makenzie B. 2016. "The Crazy Quilt of Laws: Bringing Uniformity to Surrogacy Laws in the United States." Senior Thesis, Trinity College, Hartford, Connecticut.

Ruth, Elizabeth. 2011. "Lesbian Infertility a Feminist Issue." *Herizons*.

Sallam, H. N. and N. H. Sallam. 2016. "Religious Aspects of Assisted Reproduction." *Facts Views Vis Obgyn*.

Sandel, Michael J. 2004. "The Case against Perfection." *Atlantic*.

Sarantaki, A. et al. 2015. "Families Created by In Vitro Fertilization (IVF) in Greece: Parenting Stress and Parental Bonding at Adolescence." *International Archives of Medicine, Psychiatry and Mental Health.*

Schenker, Joseph G. 2005. "Assisted Reproductive Practice: Religious Perspectives." *Reproductive BioMedicine Online.*

Scherrer, Urs et al. 2015. "Cardiovascular Dysfunction in Children Conceived by Assisted Reproductive Technologies." *European Heart Journal.*

Schuster, W. Ryan. 2016. "Rights Gone Wrong: A Case against Wrongful Life." *William and Mary Law Review.*

Scully, Jackie Leach et al. 2017. "Experiences of Faith Group Members Using New Reproductive and Genetic Technologies: A Qualitative Interview Study." *Human Fertility.*

Seifer, David B. et al. 2008. "Disparity in Assisted Reproductive Technologies Outcomes in Black Women Compared with White Women." *Fertility and Sterility.*

Selgelid, Michael J. 2015. "A Relational Approach to Saviour Siblings?" *Journal of Medical Ethics.*

Shah, Neil. 2015. "U.S. News: $30,000 Baby: There's a Lender for That— As Women Delay Having Children, Fertility-Sector Offerings Grow, from Package Deals to Loans." *Wall Street Journal.*

Shaulov, Talya et al. 2015. "Outcomes of 1503 Cycles of Modified Natural Cycle In Vitro Fertilization: A Single-Institution Experience." *Journal of Assisted Reproduction and Genetics.*

Showell, M.G. et al. 2014. "Antioxidant Vitamins and Minerals for Male Subfertility." *Cochrane Review.*

Sinclair, Daniel B. 2002. "Assisted Reproduction in Jewish Law." *Fordham Urban Law Journal.*

Slade, P. et al. 2007. "The Relationship Between Perceived Stigma Disclosure Patterns, Support and Distress in New Attendees at an Infertility Clinic." *Human Reproduction.*

Smith, Wesley J. 2011. "Savior Siblings Start Us Down Harrowing Ethical Path." *Center for Bioethics and Culture.*

Solinger, Rickie. 2013. "Reproductive Health Care Scarce for Disabled Women." www.womensenews.org.

Spar, Debora. 2007. "The Egg Trade—Making Sense of the Market for Human Oocytes." *New England Journal of Medicine.*

Speier, Amy. 2016. "A Look inside the Czech Republic's Booming Fertility Holiday Industry." *The Conversation.*

Steckler, Ashley Rae. 2016. "Finding Parenthood-Parental Identity through Assisted Reproductive Methods and the Implications for Efficacy Based and Worth Based Self-Esteem." *Cornerstone: A Collection of Scholarly and Creative Works for Minnesota State University, Mankato.*

Sultan, Aisha. 2016. "Surrogate Mom Has 3 Sets of Twins in the Past 4 Years." *St. Louis Post Dispatch.*

Svahn, M.F. et al. 2015. "Mental Disorders in Children and Young Adults among Children Born to Women With Fertility Problems." *Human Reproduction.*

Swain, Margaret E. 2016. "Assisted Reproductive Technology and the Family Law Practitioner." *American Journal of Family Law.*

Taylor-Sands, Michelle. 2010. "Saviour Siblings and Collective Family Interests." *Monash Bioethics Review.*

Thompson, Ben. 2016. "Scientists Grow Human Embryos Outside of Womb for 13 Days. Ethical?" *Christian Science Monitor.*

Tjon-Kon-Fat, R.I. et al. 2015. "Is IVF–Served Two Different Ways–More Cost-Effective Than IUI with Controlled Ovarian Stimulation?" *Human Reproduction.*

Tobias, Tamara et al. 2016. "Promoting the Use of Elective Single Embryo Transfer in Clinical Practice." *Fertility Research and Practice.*

Trifiolis, Kristie L. 2014. "Savior Siblings: The Ethical Debate." Seton Hall Law School.

U.S. Bureau of Census. 2006. https://www.myfamilymedallion.com/blog/category/blended%20family%20stats

Van Dongen, A. J. et al. 2016. "E-Therapy to Reduce Emotional Distress in Women Undergoing Assisted Reproductive Technology (ART): A Feasibility Randomized Controlled Trial." *Human Reproduction.*

Van Heesch, M. M. et al. 2015. "Hospital Costs During the First 5 Years of Life for Multiples Compared with Singletons Born after IVF or ICSI." *Human Reproduction.*

Vaughn, Rich. 2016. "Uncertain Status of Cryopreservation Agreements Creates Legal Conflict." American Bar Association.

Vera, Danielle A. 2016. "R-Egg-Ulation: A Call for Greater Regulation of the Big Business of Human Egg Harvesting." *Michigan Journal of Gender and Law.*

Verma, Shailja et al. 2016. "Pregnancy at 65, Risks and Complications." *Journal of Human Reproductive Sciences.*

Vikstrom, Josefin et al. 2017. "Risk of Postpartum Psychosis after IVF Treatment: A Nationwide Case-Control Study." *Human Reproduction.*

Vodo, Teuta. 2016. "Altruistic Surrogacy: Why to Oppose Empathetic Gestures?" *European Christian Political Movement.*

Vogel, Gretchen. 2016. "For Boys Only? Panel Endorses Mitochondrial Therapy, but Says Start with Male Embryos." *Science Magazine.*

Walker, Molly. 2016. "Some Birth Defects More Common in ART Babies." *Medpage Today OB/Gyn.*

Wallwork, Ellen. 2015. "Same-Sex Couples Could Have Babies with Genes from Both Parents Thanks to Scientific Breakthrough."*Huffpost Parents.*

Whitehead, Krista. 2016. "Motherhood as a Gendered Entitlement: Intentionality, Othering, and Homosociality in the Online Infertility Community." *Canadian Review of Sociology.*

Wilkinson, D, et al. 2015. "Double Trouble: Should Double Embryo Transfer Be Banned?". *Theories of Medical Bioethics.*

Williams, Nicola. 2016. "Should Deceased Donation Be Morally Preferred in Uterine Transplantation Trials?" *Bioethics.*

Winter, C. et al. 2015. "Psychosocial Development of Full Term Singletons, Born after Preimplantation Genetic Diagnosis (PDG) at Preschool Age and Family Function: A Prospective Case-Controlled Study and Multi-Informant Approach." *Human Reproduction.*

Wintner, Eliana M. et al. 2017. "Does the Transfer of a Poor Quality Embryo Together with a Good Quality Embryo Affect the In Vitro Fertilization (IVF) Outcome?" *Journal of Ovarian Research.*

Wong, Crystal. 2017. "In Vitro Fertilization Is Safe and Effective in SLE and APS." *Journal of Rheumatology.*

Worcester, Sharon. 2016. "Most Women Conceive within 5 Years of Starting Fertility Treatment." *Ob Gyn News.*

"World Report on Fertility Treatments Reveals High Use of Intracytoplasmic Sperm Injection." 2016. *Science Daily.*

Wright, Victoria C. et al. 2005. "Assisted Reproductive Technology Surveillance—United States, 2002." Centers for Disease Control.

Wyverkens, Elia et al. 2016. "Sister-to-Sister Oocyte Donation: Couples' Experiences with Regard to Genetic Ties." *Journal of Reproductive and Infant Psychology.*

Yeshua, Arielle et al. 2015. "Female Couples Undergoing IVF with Partner Eggs (Co-IVF): Pathways to Parenthood." *LGBT Health.*

Yildiz, M. Said and M. Mahmud Khan. 2016. "Opportunities for Reproductive Tourism: Cost and Quality Advantage of Turkey in the Provision of In-Vitro Fertilization (IVF) Services." *BMC Health Services Research.*

Ying, Liying et al. 2016. "Gender Differences in Emotional Reactions to In Vitro Fertilization Treatment: A Systematic Review."*Journal of Assisted Reproduction and Genetics.*

Yuhas, Alan and Kamala Kelkar. 2016. "Rogue Scientists Could Exploit Gene Editing Technology." *Guardian.*

Yuko, Elizabeth. 2016. "The First Artificial Insemination Was an Ethical Nightmare." *Atlantic.*

Zhang, J. J. et al. 2016. "Minimal Stimulation IVF vs Conventional IVF: A Randomized Controlled Trial." *American Journal of Obstetrics and Gynecology.*

Zinner, Susan. 2004. "Cognitive Development and Pediatric Consent to Organ Donation." *Cambridge Quarterly of Healthcare Ethics.*

Zivaridelavar, Maryam et al. 2016. "The Effect of Assisted Reproduction Treatment on Mental Health in Fertile Women." *Journal of Education and Health Promotion.*

WEBSITES

https://www.arcfertility.com/
A website dedicated to helping people choose a fertility clinic and find out which ART is appropriate for them.

https://bioethics.georgetown.edu/
Collection of bioethics resources at the Kennedy Ethical Institute at Georgetown University.

www.biomedcentral.com
Index of articles on many biological and medical subjects, including fertility.

www.bionews.org.uk
Provides news and comment on genetics, assisted conception, embryo/stem cell research and related areas.

http://buildingyourfamily.com/
Building Your Family: The Infertility and Adoption Guide
A publication and website for anyone seeking to build their family via donor egg, donor embryo, surrogacy, or adoption.

http://www.bumpstobaby.com
Bumps to Baby: A Community for Women with Infertility is a website with fertility resources and blogs.

https://www.cdc.gov/art/artdata/index.html
CDC success rates of fertility clinics in the United States.

https://www.cdc.gov/art/nass/index.html
Accessing National ART Surveillance data.

http://www.fertilityargentina.com/
Website for Argentine fertility clinic that combines fertility treatments to provide you with personal and professional attention.

http://www.fertilitypedia.org
A website hosting an Education Zone as a free resource for patients, students, and doctors. Find out about all aspects of fertility and reproductive health.

www.futuremedicine.com
Future Medicine, an imprint of Future Science Group, addresses information needs in clinical and translational medicine and the biosciences. Takes a concise and forward-looking perspective of the developments in modern health care and includes journals and eBooks that span the scientific, clinical, economic, and policy issues that confront us today.

www.givf.com
Genetics & IVF Institute
The Genetics & IVF Institute is a fully integrated, comprehensive fertility center in Fairfax, Virginia (Washington, D.C., metropolitan area). Since 1984, they have been an innovator in infertility treatment and genetics care and have helped thousands of patients worldwide realize their dreams of starting a family.

https://globalivf.com/
Medical tourism website.

https://jamanetwork.com/
Website of medical journals produced by *JAMA*.

http://www.medicaltourismassociation.com/en/index.html
Website for the Medical Tourism Association and Industry. The MTA works with healthcare providers, governments, insurance companies, employers, and other buyers of health care—in their medical tourism, international patient, and healthcare initiatives—with a focus on providing the highest quality transparent health care.

http://www.medlineplus.com
Website of medical articles, including genetics and reproduction, available at the NLM.

http://myfertilitymanual.com
A link to books, supplements, forums, and blogs about infertility and ART.

www.ncbi.nlm.nih.gov
As a national resource for molecular biology information, NCBI has the mission to develop new information technologies to aid in the understanding of fundamental molecular and genetic process that control health and disease. More specifically, the NCBI has been charged with creating automated systems for storing and analyzing knowledge about molecular biology, biochemistry, and genetics.

http://www.nyulangone.org
Websites for New York University's Langone Center with access to information on fertility.

http://www.pacificfertilitycenter.com/treatment-care/ivf/faqs
A website that shows a fertility center headed by a team of specialists guided by ethical standards and providing patients with quality, individualized, compassionate fertility care.

https://patientsbeyondborders.com/
Website on consumer information about international medical and health travel.

http://www.pewsocialtrends.org
A website that tracks the social and demographic trends in the United States, specifically the birth rate and fertility.

www.reproductivefacts.org
A website sponsored by the ASRM with information on many fertility-related topics such as insurance, fertility preservation, reproductive rights, and IVF.

www.reproductivemedicineinstitute.com
Reproductive Medicine Institute (RMI) is committed to working together to bring academic excellence, cutting-edge technology, and skilled experience in a patient-oriented practice to the Chicago area. With more than 150 years of combined experience, it has achieved unmatched success.

http://www.shinefertility.org/
Shine Fertility: A Support Group for Infertility is a website that supports women through their fertility journey by providing free mentorship, support, and education to empower and promote a proactive approach to fertility and women's health.

http://www.sistersong.net
Strengthen and amplify the collective voices of indigenous women and women of color to achieve reproductive justice by eradicating reproductive oppression and securing human rights.

MAGAZINES

BioTechniques: The International Journal of Life Science Methods
Conceive
Fertility and Sterility
IVF Lite: Journal of Minimal Stimulation
Journal of Medical Ethics
Obstetrics & Gynecology
Science News

INDEX